Vital Energy

Other Books by David Simon, M.D.

Return to Wholeness

A Simple Celebration
(with Ginna Bragg)

The Wisdom of Healing

Vital Energy

The 7 Keys to Invigorate Body, Mind, and Soul

David Simon, M.D.

John Wiley & Sons, Inc.

New York • Chichester • Weinheim • Brisbane • Singapore • Toronto

The information contained in this book is not intended to serve as a replacement for professional medical advice. Any use of the information in this book is at the reader's discretion. The author and the publisher specifically disclaim any and all liability arising directly or indirectly from the use or application of any information contained in this book. A health care professional should be consulted regarding your specific situation.

Library of Congress Cataloging-in-Publication Data:

Simon, David
    Vital energy : the 7 keys to invigorate body, mind & soul /
David Simon.
        p.   cm.
    Includes bibliographical references and index.
    ISBN 0-471-33226-7 (cloth : alk. paper)
    1. Health   2. Vitality.   3. Self-care, Health.   I. Title.
RA776.S5936   2000
613—dc21   99-28661
                                                       CIP

Printed in the United States of America
10 9 8 7 6 5 4 3 2 1

To Pam, Max, and Sara,
whose unwavering love nourishes my body, mind, and soul.

Acknowledgments

My heartfelt gratitude goes to:

Tom Miller
for your wise and gentle shepherding of this book,

Muriel Nellis and Jane Roberts
for your unfailing support,

Deepak Chopra
for your friendship and inspiration,

Eric Levine, Gayle Rose, Mallika Chopra, Sumant Chopra,
Rita Chopra, Nan Johnson, Roger Gabriel, Jenny Hathaway,
Margaret Hansley, Leanne Backer, Sandi Dean, Arielle Ford,
Debbie Ford, and Bill Elkus
for your faithful commitment to our shared dream,

Jennie Pugh and Carolyn Rangel
for your impeccability in thought, word, and deed,

and

to the entire staff of The Chopra Center for Well Being
and our worldwide IPK educators
for your ceaseless dedication to healing and transformation.

Contents

Preface

From as early as I can remember, I had a sense that I would inevitably become a doctor. I sometimes wonder if my parents whispered the suggestion into my infant ear as I was falling asleep, "You will be a doctor ... you will be a doctor ... you will be a doctor." (They assure me they did not.)

My *dharma* (purpose in life) was evident even as a child. I liked to play doctor with animals and friends in the neighborhood, and whenever an adult asked me, "What do you want to be when you grow up?" I would unhesitatingly reply, "A doctor." Physicians still made house calls while I was being raised in the suburbs of Chicago, and the esteem and affection accorded the doctor when he visited our home made a lasting impression on me.

Having this clear intention as I entered college, I wanted to understand what it really meant to be a doctor. The environment of the early seventies was a ripe time for a deeper exploration into the meaning of health and life, and so I took a step outside the usual boundaries of a premed curriculum and majored in anthropology with a focus on healing. I read everything I could find on how cultures around the world dealt with the inevitable challenges to well being and life that we all must face.

Through cross-cultural research into medicine men, shamans, and healers, I came to the understanding that the traditional role of doctor was much more than that of a disease technician. The healer was a societally sanctioned explorer into the subtle aspects of the physical, emotional, and spiritual realms of life. The doctor had to be diagnostician, medicine man, psychotherapist, and priest. Disease was viewed as a lack of integration between body, mind, and spirit, and healing was the reintegration of these layers.

The idea that illness was a purely physical event was unimaginable. In most traditional systems of health, illness begins in consciousness and the doctor must be skilled in navigating the hidden realms of existence in order to uncover and heal the imbalances, fears, and misunderstandings that give rise to disease. Even if the patient's body could not be cured of the illness, his or her soul could be healed.

Concepts of health and disease are intimately interwoven into the myths and beliefs a society holds about the natural and supernatural worlds. In most cultures, individuals were viewed as part of a cosmic web with illness representing a misalignment between personal and universal intent. The doctor's role was to identify the point of departure from balance and guide the patient back into the healthy stream of life. With an unshakable trust in the recuperative power of nature, the shaman's role was to teach— through ritual, word, and deed—the process of harmonizing the individual's body with the body of nature, the individual's mind with the mind of nature, the individual's spirit with the spirit of nature.

I learned that health and illness were the consequence of the thoughts and choices people made.

Between college and medical school, I spent several months participating in an intensive meditation course where I gained direct experience of the inner universe that is every bit as vast as the infinite outer universe. Through month after month of twelve-hour days of self-exploration, I began integrating my personal experience with the knowledge I had acquired about the body-mind-spirit connection. I began to directly experience the spectrum of environment, body, mind, and spirit that is woven to create a human being.

Entering medical school, I thought I was well prepared to begin my formal studies as a doctor: I had completed my premed requirements of biology, chemistry, and physics; had studied shamanism; and was certified to teach meditation and yoga. I actually believed that the medical community I was about to join shared my values about the importance of the body, mind, and spirit connection in the maintenance and restoration of health. I was naïve.

I remember the orientation session on my first day of medical school. Deans and professors talked about the number of Nobel

Prize winners on the faculty and how fortunate the entering class was to have been accepted to such a prestigious university. I kept listening for some hint of the sacred nature of healing that had drawn me to medicine, but was disappointed that words such as "health," "well being," "love," and "spirit" were never uttered. It seemed I was embarking upon a military career in which the enemy was disease and my job was to master the weapons to decimate the evil adversary.

I strove to master the materialistic model that permeates Western medicine, which views human beings as physical entities, knowable through an understanding of biochemistry and physiology. Awareness, thoughts, memories, desires, emotions, passion, creativity, ecstasy, and vitality are explained as byproducts of molecular and electrical interactions. In short, I learned that people are essentially physical machines that think. Peace, harmony, happiness, and love...grief, loneliness, alienation, and despair... these human experiences did not play a role in medicine, because they were not reducible to measurable elements.

This physical model of contemporary medicine is not wrong; it is merely incomplete. It has led to the phenomenal medical advances that we take for granted—coronary artery bypass surgery, cancer chemotherapy, H-2 gastric acid blockers, fourth generation antibiotics, and psychoactive medications. And yet, despite these remarkable breakthroughs in the understanding of the mechanisms of illness, modern medicine has had little impact on the expansion of well being, happiness, or vitality. We have replaced epidemics of smallpox, polio, tuberculosis, and the plague with epidemics of AIDS, heart disease, drug addiction, and cancer. We have learned a lot about how to treat illness but not much about how to create health.

My medical training taught me that health was the absence of a definable disease, and yet I have seen tens of thousands of patients who, although they are not sick, are decidedly unwell. Their laboratory studies may not demonstrate abnormalities, but the quality of their lives is far below the level they are seeking. It is in this gray zone between well being and illness that I have found the mind body approaches presented in *Vital Energy* to have tremendous value, not as a substitute for good medical treatment, but as a way to enliven the intrinsic healing forces that we all possess.

The first evidence of a decline in health is often a diminishing sense of vitality. Lack of energy, reduced enthusiasm for life, and nagging fatigue are signs that the integration between body, mind, and spirit is precarious. These days, if you go to your doctor with these complaints, you may have a series of blood tests to rule out the diseases that can sometimes cause them. Chances are very high that the tests will return normal and your physician will not be able to diagnose your problem.

When I was practicing conventional neurology, many patients with vague symptoms were referred to me to rule out neurological diseases. Rarely did I discover one. More often than not, I concluded that the person was depressed and, therefore, prescribed an antidepressant medication. I found that very frequently, some aspect of the person's condition improved, but rarely did they feel healthy or normal again. I learned that with modern medicines we can often very effectively manage people's symptoms without effecting any real healing. And with some frustration, I often found that even with an improvement in some aspect of a person's distressing symptoms, the patient did not want to continue taking the drug, because he or she wanted a deeper level of healing.

It was not until I began fully exploring the role of body, mind, and spirit in the pursuit of optimal health that I realized the most powerful healing pharmacy on earth is the human body, and there are many subtle and profound ways to enliven this inner healing system. A core message of this book is that every degradation in well being is an opportunity to identify what is missing from life so we can begin making the choices to recover the health and vitality we all deserve.

I wrote *Vital Energy* to inspire those of you who see life as a journey of self-discovery and that unlimited access to your inner ocean of vital energy is as close as your next breath. Sharing these insights with you allows me to fulfill my lifelong pursuit of becoming a doctor, for ultimately the best use of a physician's knowledge is to teach people how to heal themselves. Thank you for traveling on this path with me.

Vital Energy

Introduction

The Quest for Vitality

Truth has no special time of its own.
Its hour is now—always. —Albert Schweitzer

Quantum physicists and the perennial wisdom sages alike inform us that we are, in essence, beings of energy in a vast universe of energy. And yet if we and the entire universe are made of energy, why are so many of us tired all the time? I hear variations on the theme of this question from my patients on a daily basis. When the life force is not freely circulating, fatigue, chronic pain, weak digestion, depression, and susceptibility to infections are common. Ask your family and friends—ask yourself—do you have enough energy? Many, if not most, of the people in your life will tell you that they feel tired a lot of the time.

In a recent American study, 60 percent of people interviewed complained of fatigue in their lives. A British survey reported that one in five adults said that he or she felt tired all the time. In my daily medical practice, almost every person I see is lacking the vitality they remember or believe their life should have.

A middle-aged woman I saw in consultation recently exemplifies this concern. From all external appearances Mrs. Mason is immensely successful. She runs a flourishing marketing business, is active on several community boards, and has been married for ten years to a celebrated local attorney. She lives in a large home, drives a luxury car, and takes exotic trips at least twice a year. But despite all the accoutrements of success, Mrs. Mason is desperately unhappy and exhausted. She has been through psychological counseling and has tried several different antidepressants but continues to feel overwhelmingly tired and depleted. At work, she

1

puts up a good front but frequently finds her thoughts drifting to recurring questions in her mind: Why is she doing what she is doing? How much longer can she continue to go through the motions? What is the meaning of her life?

Although a psychiatrist might suggest that this woman's brain is deficient in serotonin, I believe that what is truly lacking is a connection with her own being. She has lost access to her vitality, her inner treasury of energy and creativity. Like so many of us, she has sought contentment in positions and possessions, but true fulfillment is impossible without clear access to vitality. Fortunately, vital energy is the core of our being, and we need only to dislodge the obstacles that are blocking its flow.

We are collectively here to remember ourselves as spiritual beings, empowered to learn, serve, and celebrate. As members of a community of souls, we have a responsibility to remind each other that our essential nature is not as flesh and blood machines but as embodied spirits, temporarily condensed as individuals. As carefree, innocent children, we experience the earth as a playground, designed for the expansion of love and happiness. Watch any child playing, regardless of culture or social status, and you will witness the life force rejoicing in its own existence. The exuberance of being alive is the reward of a deep connection to the inner wellspring of vitality. Many people have forgotten their essential nature as beings of energy, but life is a process of forgetting and remembering. As we assume the mantle of responsible adults, we envelop our spirit in layers of seriousness and sobriety. For a time, we become focused on meeting our basic needs—raising a family, reaching financial goals—surviving. But life naturally progresses through cycles, and in the suitable season, the seeds of inspiration deep within our souls inevitably begin to sprout, calling for attention and nourishment.

As I make presentations on healing and transformation around the country, I find that more and more people are resonating with the message that the essential heart of our individuality is spirit. We know it's there because many of us have had glimpses of it throughout our lives. Spirit reveals itself in many ways—as periods of a deep connectedness to a force that transcends individuality, feelings of safety while facing serious threat, a sense of hope despite genuine loss, a knowing of inner power in the midst of overwhelming challenge. The essential question we are all facing is how to access this inner state of power on a consistent basis. Among my fellow aging baby boomers, the search for spirit and meaning is taking on a new urgency as we move through midlife and wonder how many more years remain for us to experience our full potential.

Vitality Questionnaire

Take a few minutes to complete the following questionnaire to assess your current vitality level. Answer each question as honestly as possible as it applies to you right now, choosing the best of the five responses that characterizes your feelings.

	Strongly disagree	*Mostly disagree*	*Neither agree nor disagree*	*Mostly agree*	*Strongly agree*
1. I am happy and enthusiastic about my work.	0	1	2	3	4
2. I am able to express my creativity in my work.	0	1	2	3	4
3. I consider several of my coworkers to be my friends.	0	1	2	3	4
4. The people with whom I work respect me.	0	1	2	3	4
5. My work provides me opportunities for personal growth.	0	1	2	3	4
6. My most intimate relationships are nourishing.	0	1	2	3	4

	Strongly disagree	Mostly disagree	Neither agree nor disagree	Mostly agree	Strongly agree
7. I can openly communicate my feelings and needs to my family and friends.	0	1	2	3	4
8. I have people in my life whom I regularly tell I love, and who regularly say they love me.	0	1	2	3	4
9. I have people in my life whom I regularly physically touch and who touch me lovingly.	0	1	2	3	4
10. There is no one in my life that I consider to be an enemy.	0	1	2	3	4
11. My appetite and digestion are strong and healthy.	0	1	2	3	4
12. My elimination is regular and effortless.	0	1	2	3	4
13. I fall asleep easily and sleep soundly at night.	0	1	2	3	4
14. My body is free from physical pain.	0	1	2	3	4
15. I have the energy and stamina to accomplish my goals each day.	0	1	2	3	4

	Strongly disagree	Mostly disagree	Neither agree nor disagree	Mostly agree	Strongly agree
16. I am happy to be alive.	0	1	2	3	4
17. Anxiety and depression are rare experiences for me.	0	1	2	3	4
18. I genuinely like the person I am.	0	1	2	3	4
19. I feel comfortable alone and in the company of others.	0	1	2	3	4
20. I accept my strong feelings and the variety of my emotions.	0	1	2	3	4
21. I believe that there is something to be learned from every life experience.	0	1	2	3	4
22. I feel connected to my core beliefs and life mission.	0	1	2	3	4
23. I feel connected to a spiritual source.	0	1	2	3	4
24. I experience the magic and mystery of life on a regular basis.	0	1	2	3	4
25. I feel a sense of compassion for and connectedness with living beings I encounter in my life.	0	1	2	3	4
Total each column	_____	_____	_____	_____	_____
Total Vitality Score			_____		

Interpreting the Vital Energy Questionnaire

If your total vitality score is 90 points or greater, you are directly in touch with your inner vitality. My recommendation is that you give this book to a friend who needs it more than you do and continue enjoying your life.

If your score is between 75 and 90 points, you are generally in tune with your vital energy but can benefit from the reminders I'll be offering throughout this book. You have probably been overextending yourself for the last several months. Take the time to assess the imbalances that are arising in your life and realign your priorities.

If your score is between 50 and 75 points, you can probably remember a time in the not too distant past when you felt much better than you do now. Focus on the important elements that comprise your physical, emotional, and spiritual life so you can regain the energy and enthusiasm that is legitimately yours.

If your vitality score is between 25 and 50 points, you are feeling overloaded most of the time and are probably wondering when, if ever, you will feel like yourself again. Your life took a detour off your anticipated course, and you are beginning to doubt whether you will ever be able get back on track again. I see people in my practice on a daily basis who fall into this situation, and I want to assure you that with the right attention and intention, the road back home is right around the corner. This book will serve as a map for your body, mind, and soul until it becomes obvious to you that you are again on the right path.

If your vitality score is below 25 points, I know you must be struggling on a daily basis. Even the thought of making changes to improve your life may seem overwhelming. I encourage you to take small steps in the direction of greater vitality. Try one suggestion at a time for improving your well being. As you begin to notice your vital energy rising, take further steps to remove the obstacles to your rightful emotional and physical prosperity.

The Timeless Search for Vital Energy

Look around and notice the forms that surround you. I am sitting in my office at an antique hardwood desk, carved in India, assembled in Indonesia, and purchased in Los Angeles. Many years ago, it was a sapling tree, miraculously transforming the minerals of the earth, the water of the river, the carbon in the air, and light energy from our local star into roots, bark, stems, and leaves. Many years from now, long after I cease to sit here, my desk will surrender its elements back to their sources. Ten thousand years from now, a carbon atom trapped in my wooden drawer may call its home the bill of a woodpecker in southern India, hammering holes in the bark of a descendant of the tree that sacrificed its body for my desk.

The sautéed carrots in my lunch were harvested on an organic farm in Del Mar, California, less than a week ago. In its development, the carrot tapped into the energy of the sun to create vitamin A, which is liberated in my digestive tract and incorporated into the cells of my retina. The energy cycle is completed as the vibrations of sunlight, condensed in the carrot and deposited in my eyes, allow me to appreciate the rainbow arching across the morning sky.

No matter what I gaze upon, I perceive condensations of energy. The bold scientific explorers of the twentieth century illuminated the ultimate truth about the natural world. The brilliant physicists Niels Bohr, Werner Heisenberg, and Albert Einstein compelled us to look beyond the masquerade of matter and recognize the world of form in its naked state as simply energy in disguise.

The search for greater vitality is timeless. The age-old myths remind us that the search for unlimited energy and exuberance is as old as humanity. The ancient Sumerian king Gilgamesh spent his life searching for immortality. His story relates that after many perilous years he finds the secret youth-restoring plant of the gods at the bottom of the sea, only to have it stolen by a giant serpent before he is able to sample it. Alexander the Great journeyed most of his thirty-three years to the corners of the world, seeking the Well of Life, believed to be the source of waters that bestow immortality. The myth relates that Alexander's cook accidentally discovers these rejuvenative waters, but cannot remember which well he drank from, forcing the powerful conqueror to face his mortality. As schoolchildren, we learned of Ponce de León's quest for the fountain of youth in the New World. Although dense, dangerous jungles and snake-infested swamps obscured passage to this well-spring of vitality, Ponce de León was unrelenting in his efforts, spurred on by descriptions of old men regaining their vitality after a single drink.

It's fascinating how these timeless stories from around the world reflect our collective mind and reveal our fundamental universal themes. The quest for the elixir of vitality is hardwired into our consciousness. We explore the world in search of something outside ourselves, but the vital waters are not to be found in the outer world. We can spend our entire lives seeking fulfillment through our conquest, but in the end, what we are seeking lies within.

The quest for vitality is both practical and mystical. We all want sufficient energy to accomplish the mundane and grand goals of our lives. We want enough energy to work, love, learn, and enjoy life. If you are in a state of chronic exhaustion and are having trouble just doing the laundry, feeling a little more alive each day is a big accomplishment. If you are a businessperson and, despite financial success, feel your life is dry and uninspired, reconnecting with your creative source can make a dramatic change in your day-to-day reality. If you have recently been through a divorce and are feeling disoriented and alienated from yourself, getting back in touch with your core beliefs can be heartening, even exhilarating. If you are recovering from surgery or a major illness and cannot seem to get back in your groove, having days when you feel energized again can provide hope and encouragement that you are on a healing course.

On a deeper level, the pursuit of vital energy is a sacred and mystical journey. It is a soul pilgrimage that ultimately takes us to a place beyond time and space. Gilgamesh's quest for immortality, Alexander's pursuit of the Well of Life, and Ponce de León's search for the Fountain of Youth are the stories we tell that describe the inner journey of self-discovery. We are all seeking greater well being on physical, emotional, and spiritual levels. Depending upon the past and present issues in our lives, our focus may be more on one level than another. Regardless of the obstacles facing us at any stage of life, the principles for progress are universal. They are the vital energy keys we will be discovering together.

The Vital Voyage

As beautifully expressed by Marcel Proust, "The real voyage of discovery consists not in seeking new landscapes, but having new eyes." In our search for the energy and vitality we seek, we will explore the many layers that constitute human life. I have found that the most valuable framework for exploring life and health comes from *Ayurveda*, the ancient system of healing that originated in India. The roots of this profound science of life go deep into antiquity, when humankind was more directly connected to the forces of nature. Thousands of years ago, wise seers peered into their inner and outer worlds and perceived universal patterns. With these insights they created a framework for understanding life and death, health and sickness.

The recognition that human beings are inextricably woven into the fabric of nature is the essence of Ayurveda. Vitality is the fruit of the harmonious exchange of energy and information between individuals and their environment. Fatigue, unhappiness, and ultimately illness are the by-products of imbalanced, inadequate, or contaminated interactions between one's environment, body, mind, and soul. The root cause of suffering is the accumulation of unprocessed experiences from the past. The solution common to all problems is to dissolve the accumulated toxicity and allow the life force to flow from its source deep within our being to every aspect of our lives.

Ayurveda has a word for these toxins that inhibit the free flow of our life force—*ama*, a Sanskrit word that means "undigested." The concept of ama has profound implications, for it suggests that all problems are due to weak digestion. As a Western-trained medical doctor, I first scoffed at the idea that all illness stemmed from digestive disturbances. However, my initial smugness dissolved as I began to appreciate the deeper significance of this concept. Ama is not created solely from the extra piece of strawberry cheesecake that keeps us up all night with heartburn. Ama is the

by-product of anything in our lives that we do not fully metabolize at the time it is occurring. If you fail to express yourself
openly and honestly in a relationship, you accumulate ama. If you
stay in a job that brings you little satisfaction, you accumulate
ama. If you attempt to fulfill an emotional need with drugs or
food, you accumulate ama. If you resist dealing with anything
painful while it is occurring, you store the undigested pain in your
mind and body where it begins to drain your vitality. Like an infection that depletes your immune reserve, stored physical and
emotional toxins exhaust your vital energy. To rechannel the life
force that is drained by undigested residues of life-damaging experiences, ama needs to be digested on physical, mental, and emotional levels.

This book is dedicated to teaching you how to identify and
eliminate the toxic residues that are inhibiting your vital force.
We'll explore the primary facets of life—thinking, eating, loving,
working, playing, releasing. In the course of uncovering the obstacles to the spontaneous healthy functioning of our basic life
processes I will be asking you for something difficult—to be totally honest with yourself. Only in honestly assessing what is missing and what is unnecessary in our lives can we successfully bring
about the healing and transformation we seek. Confronting aspects of ourselves that we have been hiding is never easy, but it is
essential if we are to recover our vitality.

You are a unique tapestry woven together of your environment
and your senses, along with your body, mind, and spirit. As a human being you are a network of energy and information in a vast
ocean of energy and information. Together in this book we will
navigate a passageway to your field of unbounded vitality. In this
program, we'll explore seven key vitality principles. To help
enliven the vital energy principle we are exploring, vitality-
enhancing prescriptions will be introduced for each chapter.

I encourage you to focus on one key principle at a time, with
the intention of consciously and fully implementing the recommendations. The two most powerful forces in the world are your

attention and intention, and you can use these to blast away the obstacles that are inhibiting your vitality and enthusiasm. Enthusiasm is the natural state of wonder and excitement that each of us knew as children and deserves to recapture if it has been lost. It literally means "filled with spirit."

Over the course of this book you will embrace the principles and practices that will enable you to tap into your inner ocean of vital energy. A step at a time, you will reach your goal—a life abundant with vital energy.

Vital Energy Key #1

Seek Your Self

The thing we tell of can never be found seeking,
yet only seekers find it. —ABU YAZID AL-BISTAMI

Why are you the person you are? Why do you respond to situations and circumstances the way you do? Why are you attracted to certain people, places, and ideas while you are repulsed by others? What are your unique talents, and are you making the most of them? Are you living your life to the fullest extent possible?

People have been asking themselves these questions since the dawn of humankind. We all have basic needs and face similar challenges in life. To experience vibrant physical and emotional health, each of us requires fulfilling relationships, a measure of material abundance, an opportunity to express our talents in the world, and a sense of connectedness to something greater than ourselves. In Ayurveda, these basic needs are known as the Four Primary Aspirations: love, abundance, purpose, and enlightenment. Our ability to attain these life goals determines the difference between sickness or health, frustration or fulfillment, exhaustion or vitality. Only when we are in tune with our inner field of energy and creativity are we capable of achieving these aspirations with ease and joy. The best way to evaluate whether we are moving in the direction of greater well being is by listening to our inner messages of comfort or distress. Our highest evolutionary path is the one that generates the least resistance and the greatest joy.

Although people are united across time and place in seeking these four fruits of living, the history of humanity chronicles the variety of approaches to reach these essential goals. Throughout the ages, seers and sages, having experienced profound fulfillment, have offered their guidance in helping the rest of us know a greater reality. The prescriptions are remarkably similar across time and cultures. The inscription at the Delphic oracle urges us to "Know thyself." Lao-tzu reminds us, "He who knows others is wise. He who knows himself is enlightened." The Bible tells us, "Wisdom is the principal thing: Therefore get wisdom. And in all your getting, get understanding." These are nice words. How do you make them real in your daily life?

You make them real by consciously embarking on a journey of self-discovery. You need to ask the basic questions "Who am I at my core?" and "What do I really want?" By listening to your inner voice, the direction for your soul's journey will be set.

Envision a Fulfilling Life

Most people want more from their lives than they currently have. After "Mama" and "Dada," "more" is one of the first words a child learns to pronounce. Desiring more is the impulse that drives us to expand our knowledge and experiences in pursuit of greater happiness. Unfortunately, I find many of my patients wasting their valuable vital energy dwelling on what they do *not* want— dead-end jobs, loveless relationships, congested cities. In order to manifest greater vitality, you need to imagine the life that will bring you happiness. You must focus on where you want to go if you are to arrive at your goal.

Understanding your present circumstances is an important, but only a first, step in restoring vitality to life. Consider where you are, but more important, envision where you would like to be. Notice what is getting in the way of achieving your goals, and recognize that most obstacles are due to disempowering beliefs rather than insurmountable external forces. Begin the process now of creating a life rich in vital energy by working through the following exercises.

1. On a scale of 1 (low) to 10 (high), honestly rate your current level of fulfillment in each of these four areas of life:

Love   _____

Material abundance   _____

Purpose in life   _____

Spiritual fulfillment   _____

2. As honestly as possible, describe what is getting in the way of your fulfilling your aspirations.

Love (Example: I am not creating the fulfilling relationships I seek because I am overly critical of other people's imperfections. I hold unachievable standards of perfection for myself and others and therefore am often disappointed.)

_____

_____

_____

_____

_____

_____

Material abundance (Example: I am not achieving the material abundance I seek because I keep hoping that good luck will compensate for my lack of discipline.)

_____

_____

_____

_____

_____

_____

Purpose in life (Example: I am not establishing myself in a role that brings me fulfillment because what I really want to do has never received the support of those from whom I seek approval.)

_____

_____

_____

_____

_____

_____

Spiritual fulfillment (Example: I am not taking time to explore my spiritual development because I am afraid of losing favor with my current circle of relationships, which doesn't support contemplative or philosophical approaches to life.)

_____

_____

_____

_____

_____

_____

3. Describe what more you can do to enhance the fulfillment of each aspiration.

Love (Example: I will practice nonjudgment, seeking to appreciate the different ways people view life, rather than trying to impose my perspective on everyone around me.)

_____

_____

_____

_____

_____

_____

Material abundance (Example: I will live within a budget that balances my needs in the present with my goals for the future. I will allocate a portion of my time and energy to create the future I envision, and be alert to my tendency to fulfill my emotional needs with material objects.)

_____

_____

_____

_____

_____

_____

Purpose in life (Example: I will pursue a vision of life that derives from my innermost desires. I will develop my unique abilities and trust that my commitment to work that is fulfilling will generate material abundance.)

_____

_____

_____

_____

_____

Spiritual fulfillment (Example: I will set aside quiet time in my busy schedule. I will relinquish the need for others' approval of my desire to explore my inner resources.)

_____

_____

_____

_____

_____

From the very beginning I encourage you to get into the habit of writing down your responses rather than simply contemplating them in your mind. Start a journal, and take time each day to make entries. For these exercises, silently ask yourself the questions and listen to the quiet voice within you for the answers. Many people find the best time to journal is before they go to bed. If you create the time and space to record your inner dialogue, you will soon begin to see your intentions and desires manifesting themselves in your life.

Making Vital Energy Real

Imagine Fulfillment

1. Allow time in your day to consider what you want in your life that will bring you greater vitality, love, and happiness.
2. Set your sights on a life vision that fulfills your physical, emotional, and spiritual needs. Make choices that move you in the direction of achieving your goals.
3. Focus on what you want in your life, not on what you don't want. Do not waste your vital energy lamenting the results of your past choices. Channel your life force into avenues that allow you to fulfill your deepest aspirations.

Tune In to the Wisdom of Life

The word *Ayurveda* means "wisdom of life." Wisdom is the integration of understanding and experience. Ayurveda provides the keys to both, viewing people as woven from the fabric of the natural world and offering a process to reestablish access to the vital forces of nature. With a little adaptation, the thousand-year-old formulas of Ayurveda are vibrantly relevant to modern times. To tap into the power of the universe, we need to understand the integral role we play in the cosmos. The same forces responsible for the movement of galaxies and the blossoming of a rose govern the birth of a child and the genesis of our thoughts. The more unimpeded our connection to this underlying field of intelligence, the more energy, joy, and abundance flow in our lives.

Look around you and imagine that you are the first person to try to make sense of the natural world. What is the world made of? You see solid structures made from the earth that maintain their mass and shape over time. You observe water that has substance but no shape of its own and see how it carries other things as it flows. You experience the heat and light of the sun or the flames in your fireplace and observe the powerful transformational effect of fire. You notice the motion of air, invisible and without structure, yet capable of moving earth, water, and fire. And between objects you perceive the eternal emptiness of space within which the other elements reside. According to Ayurveda you have elaborated the five fundamental codes of nature: mass, fluidity, transformation, movement, and expansion. Anything that we can perceive can be known in terms of these basic forces.

We tend to forget that we are part of nature, made of the same stuff that comprises a distant star, a majestic mountain, or a towering redwood tree. We too have these primary forces dancing within. When these elements are harmonious, we feel vital. When they are discordant, we feel fatigue. Understanding our natural state of balance and honestly assessing where we have gone awry are essential steps toward optimum vitality.

The Three Vital Elements

We can make the five primary forces of nature even simpler when applying them to living systems. Matter, metabolism, and motion are the three fundamental principles that govern our lives. The matter, or material, principle is known in Ayurveda as *Kapha*. Our muscles, bones, organs, and tissues are essentially different types of matter mixed together with water. The cell, the fundamental building block of our anatomy, is a watery bag of protein and salt bound up with sugars, fats, and a smattering of other chemicals. The matter of our body is formed from the raw material we ingest from our environment. If the morsels we consume are nourishing, we create a healthy, vital body. If not, we pay the consequences with ill health and fatigue. To make it easy to remember, we'll call our vital matter element *Earth*, for like the earth our bodies are made of solid and liquid forms of matter.

The metabolism principle governs transformation in living systems. The conversion of food into tissues and energy, the digestion of new ideas, and the processing of emotions are all different forms of transformation. When your digestive powers are strong and vibrant, you are capable of metabolizing any input into your mind or body and deriving the energy and information you need. The Ayurvedic term for the metabolism principle is *Pitta*, but we will refer to it as *Fire*.

The motion element is responsible for all movement within your mind and body. The motion principle governs the movement of thoughts, breath, muscles, and circulating blood as well as the movement of food through your digestive tract. Known in Ayurveda as *Vata*, we will call the movement principle *Wind*, for like the wind, the movement force can propel matter and fan the fire of metabolism.

Earth, Fire, and Wind are the elements of the universe and of your personal biology. The more intimate you become with them on physical, emotional, and mental planes, the more easily you can use these fundamental forces to create vitality in your life. Understanding the world in terms of these three elementary principles is easy and fun. It simply requires shifting your perspective and directing your attention and intention.

Making Vital Energy Real

Earth, Fire, and Wind Scenarios

Spend today considering your world in terms of the three primary principles of Earth, Fire, and Wind. Notice how different combinations and permutations of the basic forces of matter, transformation, and motion govern your daily activities and responses. When something unanticipated happens during your day today, reflect on which of the three forces is expressing itself.

As examples, consider the following situations and identify which of the primary forces, Earth, Fire, or Wind, is at work.

1. _____ Your car overheats.

2. _____ You feel heavy and dull after a big meal.

3. _____ Your racing mind keeps you from falling asleep at night.

4. _____ You get heartburn after eating spicy food.

5. _____ You feel gassy and bloated after eating cabbage soup.

6. _____ You get sunburned at the beach.

7. _____ You get nasal congestion after eating a bowl of ice cream.

8. _____ You have a heated argument with a coworker.

9. _____ Your heart beats rapidly as you drive to a job interview.

10. _____ Your term paper flies out the window of your car.

Notice how this simple perspective helps to make sense out of a complex world.

ANSWERS:				
1. Fire	2. Earth	3. Wind	4. Fire	5. Wind
6. Fire	7. Earth	8. Fire	9. Wind	10. Wind

Understand Your Mind Body Nature

We all embody these three basic principles to varying degrees. The Earth principle creates, supports, and lubricates our cells and tissues. The Fire principle governs the ongoing metamorphosis of food into cells and cells into waste, and the generation of energy required to carry out the many activities we perform in a day. The Wind principle ensures that our DNA strands zip and unzip, that vital gases flow in out and of cells, and that nerve impulses travel from head to toe and back again. These forces are continually dancing with each other, directing the vital force to and through every cell in the body. When they are functioning in harmony, the dance of life is elegant beyond words. When they are out of sync, fatigue, stress, distress, and disease arise.

These forces are present in all of us. But what makes me different from you? What makes each of us special? The answer has to do with how we have uniquely woven these three fundamental principles into the fabric of our mind body network. We all integrate our experiences with propensities to express a particular mind body constitution. My experiences have been different from yours, but even if they had been similar, I would be different from you because my inherited proportions of Earth, Fire, and Wind are different from yours. Ayurveda recognizes that both nature and nurture play important roles in creating the person you are. Applying modern terminology to this timeless knowledge, we could say that through our parents' DNA we inherit our relative proportions of the three primary elements, and then influence their expression through our life experiences. Let's see if we can characterize your nature according to these principles.

Determine Your Mind Body Nature: A Questionnaire

I would like you to take the following questionnaire designed to help you determine your true mind body nature. To complete this first set of questions, bring to mind a time in your life when you were your healthiest and happiest. This may be now, or some time in the recent past. You may have to think back to your childhood to identify your most vibrant and vital phase. Take a minute or two to recall as clearly as possible a time when you felt most alive. When this image is vivid in your awareness, rate yourself on each of the following questions as honestly as possible. Don't spend more than a few moments considering your response. Circle the answer that first comes to mind. Remember, these questions are designed to determine your inherent nature at a time when you were not so encumbered by the stresses and challenges that may be weighing on you now. There are no right or wrong responses, so simply answer the questions as truthfully as you can.

Your Mind Body Nature Questionnaire

SECTION 1	not me at all	me to some extent	definitely me
1. I am a nurturing person.	1	3	5
2. I sleep deeply.	1	3	5
3. I am steady and methodical.	1	3	5
4. I am sturdy.	1	3	5
5. I am forgiving.	1	3	5
6. I have large bones.	1	3	5
7. I am a good listener.	1	3	5
8. I have good skin.	1	3	5
9. My digestion is smooth and regular.	1	3	5
10. I am easygoing.	1	3	5

Section 1 Score _____

SECTION 2	not me at all	me to some extent	definitely me
1. I am smart.	1	3	5
2. I like to lead.	1	3	5
3. I do not need much sleep.	1	3	5
4. I have a strong appetite.	1	3	5
5. I am goal-oriented.	1	3	5
6. I value punctuality.	1	3	5
7. I like to win.	1	3	5
8. I am discriminating.	1	3	5
9. I stand up for my beliefs.	1	3	5
10. I like cool weather.	1	3	5

Section 2 Score _____

SECTION 3	not me at all	me to some extent	definitely me
1. I have a quick mind.	1	3	5
2. I am always on the move.	1	3	5
3. I sleep lightly.	1	3	5

SECTION 3 *(cont.)*	*not me at all*	*me to some extent*	*definitely me*
4. I am thin.	1	3	5
5. I am enthusiastic.	1	3	5
6. I do not like routines.	1	3	5
7. I am a lively conversationalist.	1	3	5
8. I eagerly take on new projects.	1	3	5
9. I like change.	1	3	5
10. I prefer warm weather.	1	3	5

Section 3 Score _____

MIND BODY *NATURE SCORE*

Section 1 (Earth) _____
Section 2 (Fire) _____
Section 3 (Wind) _____

Interpreting Your Scores

Look at your Earth, Fire, and Wind scores from this questionnaire, ranking them in order from highest to lowest. This order
tells you the relative ranking of these primordial forces in your nature. If you scored highest in the Fire category, with lower scores
in Earth and Wind, you have primarily a fiery nature. If your two
highest scores are within five points of each other, such as Wind
and Fire, then both of these elements are fairly equally represented. Rarely, all three scores fall within five points of each other,
which suggests that all three forces are evenly represented in your
mind body physiology. There are seven basic mind body types described by this system:

- Primarily Earth
- Primarily Fire
- Primarily Wind
- Earth and Fire (or Fire and Earth)

- Earth and Wind (or Wind and Earth)
- Fire and Wind (or Wind and Fire)
- Earth, Fire, and Wind

The 7 Mind Body Types

Let's characterize each of the seven possible constitutions in more detail. As I describe the classic features of each mind body type, see how closely your traits align themselves with the characteristics of the constitutional type determined from your questionnaire scores.

EARTH TYPE (Your Earth score is more than 5 points higher than the next-highest element). Emily was the eldest of four children. Even as a child, she had a nurturing instinct. She tended to carry a few extra pounds since her preteen years but was well liked by her peers for her reliability and loyalty. As an adult she married young and enjoyed raising her own family. She was known for her baking talent, which she sampled regularly herself. By the time she reached forty, she was pushing 180 pounds and showing evidence of mildly elevated blood pressure. When her mother became ill with breast cancer, Emily fulfilled the expectations of her siblings, assuming the role of primary caregiver. It was not until after her mother had completed her course of treatment that Emily began to notice how tired she was much of the time. Despite the fact that she was sleeping more than usual, she had trouble getting going in the morning, and her weight became even more difficult to control because she was less active.

According to Ayurveda, Emily has a natural predominance of the Earth element in her nature, which has become increasingly imbalanced. To regain access to her inner reservoir of vital energy, she needs to follow an invigorating diet and lifestyle, allowing time for daily self-nurturing.

If your highest score is in the Earth category, your nature is steady, easygoing, and tolerant. You are connected to the earth and tend to be careful, patient, and forgiving. Physically you may be stocky, with a tendency toward being overweight. You may complain that you only need to look at a piece of cheesecake and you put on a pound. Your daily habits tend to be methodical without being obsessive. You go to bed at about the same time each night and awaken with an alarm clock in the morning. You tend to be slower in the early hours and, given the chance, love to sleep in. You try to avoid confrontation and conflict whenever possible, and you are often the peacemaker in your family and at work. When your feelings are hurt, you usually withdraw and try to disguise your pain. You are much more comfortable taking care of others than having your own needs fulfilled. You tend to accumulate stuff and have difficulty letting go of things, emotions, and people, even if they are no longer nourishing you. When you are in balance, you are sweet, dependable, even-tempered, and loyal. When you get out of balance, you tend to withdraw to the point of hibernation, padding yourself physically and emotionally from the perceived sources of pain in your life.

FIRE TYPE (Your Fire score is more than 5 points higher than the next-highest element). Kenneth was always ambitious by nature. He liked to compete and liked to win. After completing law school he became a litigator in a major New York firm, developing a successful career and gaining a reputation as a fierce opponent. At home he was warm and loving with his children but tended to be controlling about money with his wife. Shortly after losing a major product liability case, he began having regular throbbing headaches. When simple over-the-counter pain relievers failed to relieve his pain, his physician diagnosed migraines. Although usually able to bulldoze his way through challenges, Kenneth found it increasingly difficult to regain his drive after these emotional and physical assaults on his sense of invulnerability. He felt he was on the verge of burnout.

From an Ayurvedic perspective, Kenneth is demonstrating symptoms of imbalance in his inherently fiery constitution. He needs to learn how to cool off the excessive heat in his mind and body with relaxation time, diet, and activities. Left unchecked, he is at risk of irreversibly scorching his body, mind, and relationships.

When the Fire element is predominant in your nature, you are intense, with a strong appetite for the world. You are passionate and enjoy the finer things in life. Looking good and making a good impression on others are important to you. You have a sharp intellect that helps you make fine discriminations. You can be a good debater and pride yourself on not compromising when you hold a strong belief about something. Physically you have a medium build with good muscle development. You enjoy eating, have a strong digestion, and tend toward loose elimination, particularly when you are under stress. You enjoy working on a project and feel that you are wasting time if you are not directing your efforts toward a goal. You are purposeful and competitive. When your life is in balance, you are a good leader, a warm friend, and articulate. When you get overheated, you can be argumentative and intimidating.

WIND TYPE (Your Wind score is more than 5 points higher than the next-highest element). Sharon was always the life of the party. Friendly and outgoing, she was never at a loss for words and thrived on being the center of attention. Throughout high school and college, she moved through a series of relationships, preferring to play the field rather than getting serious with one person. Although she did well in her college classes if she applied herself, she tended to get by on charm rather than academic competence and changed her major several times before deciding on advertising. Once in the work world, she got bored easily with each position and made mostly lateral moves when she changed jobs. Her history of personal relationships was similarly restless, with her first marriage lasting just over a year and her second dissolving shortly after she decided that she needed to change coasts to take a new job.

It wasn't until her mid-thirties that she began to notice that her energy level was not what it used to be. She was sleeping poorly at night, and her digestion was increasingly delicate. Her usual enthusiasm for new adventures had faded, and she developed a sense of underlying anxiety and subtle depression.

According to Ayurveda, her underlying Wind propensity has progressed to a Wind imbalance. She needs physical, emotional, and spiritual grounding in order to reconnect with her vital energy source.

When the movement principle is dominant in your physiology, your nature is lively and enthusiastic. You like to engage other people and enjoy conversation. Routine does not appeal to you. You tend to go to sleep, wake up in the morning, and eat your meals at varying times from one day to the next. You are open to new experiences and are generally better at starting new projects or programs than following through with them. You have an active and creative mind and become restless unless you are on the move. Physically you tend to be thin and lanky. You may not have a strong appetite, and your digestion can be delicate. When your life is balanced, you are vivacious, dynamic, and spirited. When under stress, you get out of balance, your movement tendencies become exaggerated, and your mind and body become turbulent and unsettled.

In addition to the three primary mind body constitutions, you can have a nature that has strong features of more than one type. Most people do not have pure Earth, Fire, or Wind natures, but relatively higher proportions of two elements compared to the third. A very few people are equally balanced in all three mind body energies. An awareness of how your mind body components interact will help you understand your nature and tendencies at a subtler level and make corrections if you move too far out of balance.

EARTH-FIRE or FIRE-EARTH (Your Earth and Fire scores are within 5 points of each other, and both are greater than the Wind score). When both Earth and Fire are well represented, you are likely to be powerful and successful. Your fiery nature drives you, while your earthiness keeps your grounded and provides you with the endurance to accomplish your goals. You are a good leader who is both respected and appreciated. You have a strong appetite, which predisposes you to gain weight, but you can usually muster the discipline to work it off when you find yourself tipping the scales above where you want to be. You may be a good athlete and enjoy recreational activities and friendly competitive sports. It takes a lot to exhaust you, but if you chronically overextend yourself, you can spend an entire weekend catching up on your sleep. You do not become upset easily, but once you do, it takes a long time for you to forgive and forget.

EARTH-WIND or WIND-EARTH (Your Earth and Wind scores are within 5 points of each other, and both are greater than the Fire score). The Earth and Wind elements generally express opposite qualities. Earth creates stability; Wind generates change. Earth tends toward heaviness and supports routine; Wind governs lightness and spontaneity. When these two principles are prominent in your nature, these inwardly and outwardly directed forces are challenging to balance. Earth and Wind are united by their tendency to produce coldness, and people with Earth-Wind constitutions often have a lack of heat in their mind body nature. You may look as if you physically have an Earth constitution with a large frame and a tendency to gain weight, yet your mind is likely to be active and creative. When you are under stress, you will have a tendency to eat more in an effort to soothe your anxiety, which has the effect of increasing your bulk. You tend to be a sweet and forgiving person who is uncomfortable expressing hot emotions such as anger or passion. Earth-Wind people benefit from bringing more heat into their lives.

FIRE-WIND or WIND-FIRE (Your Fire and Wind scores are within 5 points of each other, and both are greater than the Earth score). Wind added to Fire can generate a lot of heat or can extinguish the flames altogether. If Wind and Fire are the predominant elements in your nature, you are dynamic and intense. You can be very passionate, although your staying power may be somewhat limited. You will tend to have a strong appetite but not necessarily a large capacity. Your physique tends toward the lean and wiry.

Your mind can race, thinking about all the things you need to accomplish. You like to move, as long as it is in the direction of a goal you have set. When you are balanced, you have a voracious capacity for learning new things, which you easily master. When you become out of balance due to the stresses of life, you can become testy, whiny, cynical, and biting.

EARTH-WIND-FIRE (All three scores are within 5 points of each other). This pattern is the rarest of the mind body constitutions. If matter, metabolism, and motion are fairly equally represented in your nature, you are balanced and adaptable. In your emotional life you experience a range of feelings without allowing yourself to get too dramatic. Your physical health is generally good, with your nature reflecting the qualities present in your environment. During the cold, wet season, your Earth qualities are more readily apparent. During the hot summer months, your Fire traits are more likely to be expressed. During the cold, blustery winter season, your Wind characteristics may arise. Staying in balance for you means paying attention to your environment and adjusting accordingly. If you have accumulated imbalances in all three elements, it usually means that you have amassed an excessive amount of toxicity. We'll explore how to clear your system of toxins in the next chapter.

Making Vital Energy Real

Know Your Nature

As you characterize the predominant forces in your mind and body, begin to witness the patterns that underlie your emotional and physical reactions. Observe your responses to challenges in your life and witness how your underlying nature expresses the three primary forces of movement, transformation, and stability. Notice how your mind body constitution governs your tendencies. Before you go to sleep each night, record a situation or circumstance that you recognize as expressing a prominent quality of Earth, Fire, or Wind.

As an example—

Situation: When picking up my laundry at the dry cleaner's, I noticed a button was missing. When the clerk did not respond as respectfully as I expected, I became irritated and chastised him sarcastically.

Element expressed: My Fire element was building all day at work. It became overheated and flared up at the dry cleaner's.

Your experience:
Situation:

_____

_____

_____

Element expressed:

_____

_____

_____

Find and Understand Your Imbalance Score

In this next questionnaire, I would like you to answer each question according to how you have been feeling lately. For this test to be helpful, you need to respond as accurately and honestly as possible. Try not to filter your responses. Simply choose the answer that most closely applies to your current situation.

SECTION 1	not me at all	me to some extent	definitely me
1. I have been sleeping a lot.	1	3	5
2. I am overweight.	1	3	5
3. I eat even when I am not hungry.	1	3	5
4. I accumulate things I don't need.	1	3	5
5. I have sinus congestion or allergies.	1	3	5

	not me at all	me to some extent	definitely me
6. I have trouble ending a relationship that is not nourishing.	1	3	5
7. I have difficulty expressing my feelings.	1	3	5
8. I feel safest when I am alone.	1	3	5
9. I feel sluggish after meals.	1	3	5
10. I am excessively tolerant.	1	3	5

Section 1 Score _____

SECTION 2

	not me at all	me to some extent	definitely me
1. I have heartburn or indigestion.	1	3	5
2. I have been feeling irritable.	1	3	5
3. There are not enough hours in my day.	1	3	5
4. I am driven.	1	3	5
5. I lose my temper.	1	3	5
6. I am always hungry.	1	3	5
7. I overheat easily, even when people around me are cool.	1	3	5
8. I am argumentative.	1	3	5
9. I am perceived as controlling.	1	3	5
10. I hurt people's feelings.	1	3	5

Section 2 Score _____

SECTION 3

	not me at all	me to some extent	definitely me
1. I worry a lot of the time.	1	3	5
2. My appetite is inconsistent.	1	3	5
3. I have insomnia.	1	3	5
4. I am having trouble completing things.	1	3	5
5. I am restless.	1	3	5
6. I have been going to bed late.	1	3	5
7. I don't eat at regular times.	1	3	5
8. My bowels are unreliable.	1	3	5
9. My mind races.	1	3	5
10. I feel cold much of the time.	1	3	5

Section 3 Score _____

```
┌─────────────────────────────────────────────────────────┐
│              MIND BODY IMBALANCE SCORES                    │
│                                                            │
│   Section 1 (Earth)    _____                        │
│   Section 2 (Fire)     _____                        │
│   Section 3 (Wind)     _____                        │
│                                                            │
└─────────────────────────────────────────────────────────┘
```

Interpreting Your Mind Body Imbalance Scores

Review your scores from the second questionnaire and see in which sections you scored higher than 25 points. A perfect score of 10 for a section suggests the principle is functioning without strain, while a score of 50 warns of an impending meltdown. Any score over 30 points should be viewed as a cautionary signal that important basic areas of your life need attention. Usually, but not always, the mind body principle that is most highly represented in your healthy nature is the one that most easily moves out of balance. For example, if the Wind element is most prominent in your nature, your are most likely to find that the Wind becomes increasingly turbulent when your life is overly stressful. If Fire is most represented in your nature, you are likely to get increasingly overheated, mentally and physically, when you are overloaded. If the Earth element represents the largest part of your nature, you will tend to get heavier and more withdrawn under stress. Let's look more closely at the ways we can lose our balance according to these basic principles, so we can gain the insight necessary to recover and maintain our spiritual, emotional, and physical equilibrium.

Too Much Gravity: Earth Out of Balance

Earth types are generally appreciated by family, friends, and coworkers. When the Earth element is in balance, you provide the stability and reliability that we all cherish in a relationship. The risks for Earth types are the tendencies to accumulate too much and become too dense. Psychologically, people with a predominance of the Earth element have difficulty letting go, even when they know that they are holding on to something that is not serving them well. Relationships, jobs, and ideas whose times have long since exceeded their value remain in the lives of Earth people because of their resistance to change. I most often see this picture in nurturing women who give to the point of depletion in relationships and still feel guilty that they are considering their own needs. Children and spouses welcome the willingness of Earth mothers to give selflessly, but this pattern also has a tendency to encourage dependency that stunts self-sufficiency and independence.

I saw a woman recently who displayed these classic Earth tendencies. Patty was the rock of the family whom everyone turned to whenever they had a problem. She was always ready to sacrifice her own needs to fulfill those of others. When her husband of twenty years decided to go off with his secretary, Patty saw no choice but to assume more responsibility for the support of her three teenage children. She took on a full-time job, while still trying to keep up with the shopping, cooking, and cleaning. Despite no obvious changes in her diet, she began putting on weight and, within six months, had gained thirty pounds. She found she was talking more to herself and less to her children, while feeling continually exhausted. On weekends she stayed in bed until noon. When she visited her doctor and learned that her blood sugar was elevated, she decided it was time to do something to regain her life.

The Earth principle keeps us grounded. It stabilizes mind and body and provides lubrication over the rough spots. Without enough Earth in your system, you will feel unstable and vulnerable to the winds of change. With too much Earth in your system, you will experience sluggishness, dullness, and inertia. When the Earth principle accumulates excessively, you feel as if you have landed on a planet with much greater gravity than you are accustomed to. Everything takes more effort to accomplish, and things seem to move in slow motion. People who have accumulated disproportionate Earth in their system usually complain of feeling too heavy. They may have gained weight that they are unable to shed, feel they are retaining fluid, and often have a sense of congestion in body and mind. Allergies, bronchitis, sinus problems, obesity, diabetes, daytime drowsiness, excessive sleepiness, and generalized weakness are some of the health concerns associated with an Earth imbalance. Fibrocystic breasts and benign tumors such as uterine fibroids are also traditional manifestations of an overabundant Earth element.

The lack of vitality experienced when the Earth principle has excessively accumulated is caused by too much matter in the system, which usually results from having ingested immoderate amounts of sensory things that have a heavy, dulling effect on mind and body. Too much rich food, too much meat, too much alcohol, too many drugs, too much watching television, too much withdrawal to avoid confrontation, too much routine, too much inactivity—all these excesses can lead to the accumulation of Earth if your intake exceeds your capacity to metabolize. When our digestive system is overloaded, we lose the ability to extract what is nourishing and eliminate the surplus. We store the excess, adding to the viscosity that restricts the free flow of energy and information within our physiology. If you have amassed too much Earth, you may feel that you are moving through molasses.

Geologic time passes more slowly than biological time and people with Earth constitutions move at their own pace. They provide a steady beat and can be stabilizing for others in a frenetic world, but they can also be exasperating for other people who are inclined to respond rapidly to change and challenge. Earth types tend to be the last to finish their meals, still working on their main course while Wind types are finishing their dessert. The Earth type is usually the last one in the family to get into the car and takes the longest to get ready in the morning. Balanced, Earth types help remind us to be in the present moment. Out of balance, they can feel like driving with the emergency brake on.

Understanding the problem of excessive Earth retention opens the door to the solution. As we'll be exploring in subsequent chapters, if your Earth principle is creating too much gravity for you, the key to greater vitality is to lighten up. Lighter foods, sounds, sensations, relationships, and herbs can help dilute the density and get the energy flowing again.

Balanced Earth generates:	Imbalanced Earth generates:	To balance the Earth element:
Stability	Heaviness	Follow a lighter diet
Reliability	Sluggishness	Change your daily routine
Tolerance	Congestion	Exercise vigorously

Raging Inferno: Fire Out of Balance

Fire types drive change. Mental fire creates powerful visions, and physical fire provides the energy to manifest desires. Heads of successful entrepreneurial businesses, football quarterbacks, political and organizational leaders, and dedicated research scientists all have strong fiery natures, driving them to digest the world. Balanced, they are our best leaders, but out of balance, they can incinerate themselves and those around them. Time can be their best friend or worst enemy. Fire types measure themselves by how much they can achieve in the shortest possible time. When they are able to navigate obstacles without missing a beat, they become exhilarated and inspiring. When they are at risk of not meeting a deadline, their minds and bodies overheat and aggravation, irritation, and intimidation flare. I recently saw a man who exemplified the best and worst aspects of a fiery constitution.

Peter was a powerhouse. Shortly after joining a major investment house, he distinguished himself by his brilliance and unrelenting dedication. As his client base expanded, his sense of timing and an unrelenting bull stock market made him a confident, wealthy, and respected financial advisor. But as American businesses responded to the economic crisis in Asia, the stresses at work began taking their toll both physically and emotionally. He was so testy at the office that his assistants started calling him "the dragon man" behind his back. His irritability extended to his home life, where his temper alienated his wife and children. By the time he went to see his family physician for his heartburn, he was chewing his way through several rolls of antacid tablets each day. Because his laboratory studies suggested a mild anemia, Peter was referred to a gastroenterologist who diagnosed a bleeding peptic ulcer. He had to make some changes in his life.

The Fire element is essential for digesting the world. The principle of metabolism enables us to break down any input, be it food, words, emotions, sights, sounds, or sensations, into its elemental components. With fire we absorb the morsels we consider nourishing and leave the waste products behind. If you have a balanced fiery constitution, you are capable of digesting your environment and extracting the information, energy, and nourishment you need. If your Fire element has become aggravated because of excessive stress in your life, the heat that arises generates inflammation and irritability. Your warmth and intensity escalate to overheating and anger. Frustration, sarcasm, and intimidation arise as your internal mind body temperature mounts. Your strong appetite and powerful digestion cross the line to heartburn and acid indigestion. Your sharp intellect becomes critical, your can-do attitude becomes compulsive, and your good leadership skills begin to feel more like domination. Your blood pressure rises, and your migraine headaches recur. Time becomes the instrument by which you measure your life, and there never seems to be enough of it. Eventually, if you do not take steps to reestablish balance, you burn out. Along the way you feel escalating frustration and irritability while alienating coworkers and family members.

The key to preventing the harmful effects of aggravated Fire is to chill out. We'll explore ways to cool off your mind and body through food, massage, exercise, aromas, and herbs. The only truly effective way to conquer time-bound awareness is to embrace the present moment and stop fighting the evolutionary flow of nature by trying to force things to ripen before their time. We'll talk about how to do this in subsequent chapters.

Balanced Fire generates:	Imbalanced Fire generates:	To balance the Fire element:
Intelligence	Belittling tendencies	Focus on instruction, not destruction
Strong digestive power	Indigestion	Reduce spicy, salty, and sour foods
Goal orientation	Compulsivity	Practice better time management

Turbulent Skies: Wind Out of Balance

We live in an accelerating society. Movement and change are essential components of modern life. Motion channeled in an evolutionary direction generates progress, but motion without objective is turbulence. Although we may have forgotten that progress requires periods of rest and activity, our bodies pay the toll for ignoring the eternal rhythms of nature. A woman who recently consulted me illustrates a common scenario. Alice was a perpetual motion machine who loved attention and liked to talk. Like a hummingbird, she moved from one new project to the next, continually on the lookout for something new and exciting. She had been in and out of many passionate but short-lived relationships and was being pressured by her latest love to make a commitment. Although she knew she wasn't ready to get married, she didn't want to be alone at this time in her life. She unconsciously started skipping meals and getting to bed later. Her irritable bowel syndrome flared and she was having trouble sleeping at night.

The principle of movement is the force behind all change. If the Wind element is predominant in your nature and you are in balance, you are a person of dynamism in body and mind. Unfortunately, more than either Earth or Fire, the Wind element readily moves off balance because it is always in motion. If the challenges of life cause your Wind principle to become imbalanced, a pleasant breeze can become a cyclone. When the movement principle becomes excessive, your mind races, your body becomes restless, and agitation stirs. Wind has the effect of drying the system, so an early sign of a Wind imbalance is dryness—dry skin, dry hair, dry emotions. The turbulence of a Wind imbalance shows up in the digestive tract with variable appetite, weak digestion, and a tendency toward constipation. Pain syndromes such as tension headaches or fibromyalgia are often expressions of a Wind imbalance. The motion principle has a self-perpetuating tendency: excessive mental turbulence leads to insomnia, which exacerbates the mental and physical unrest.

Wind people have difficult relationships with time. When they are engaged in something they find fascinating, they lose track of time. When things are too routine or predictable, they become bored and time slows to a crawl. They are more often late than punctual for a meeting because they'd rather apologize for their tardiness than waste time waiting. Good friends of Wind people expect them to be late and adapt accordingly. Strong Fire types, on the other hand, often find their heat rising by the time the Wind blows in.

Counteracting the turmoil of aggravated motion requires the introduction of calming, warming, lubricating influences. Warm, heavier foods, soothing massages, a regular daily routine, and quieting herbs can all be useful tools in returning the movement principle to its healthy role in your life. Untreated, excessive Wind leads to exhaustion, anxiety, and depression. Balanced and channeled, Wind enlivens vitality.

Balanced Wind generates:	Imbalanced Wind generates:	To balance the Wind element:
Enthusiasm	Anxiety	Follow a regular daily routine
Creativity	Ungroundedness	Perform a daily oil massage
Flexibility	Irregularity	Practice goal setting

Making Vital Energy Real

Focus on Balance

Pay attention to the expressions of your mind body nature when you are comfortable and secure, as well as when you feel stressed. Notice how the same qualities within your nature can create success and happiness when you are feeling balanced or generate frustration and distress when you are off balance. If the Wind element is your dominant force, notice how lively and enthusiastic you are when you are feeling comfortable, but how anxious and erratic you become when you are stressed. If you are fiery by nature, notice how competently you are able to digest everything in your life when you are balanced, but how irritable and overheated you become when you encounter obstacles. If Earth is your predominant element, pay attention to how your normally stable and forgiving nature becomes possessive and withdrawn under stress, and how you find yourself holding on too tightly, when letting go gracefully may be the best approach. Whenever you feel physically or emotionally uncomfortable, consider the situation in terms of balance and imbalance.

Record examples of your mind body nature expressing the qualities of the elements in a balanced and imbalanced manner. Become conscious of the situations and circumstances that push you off balance.

Balanced expression

_____

_____

_____

Imbalanced expression

_____

_____

_____

Choose Your Reality

Your day-to-day reality is not merely what happens out there; your reality is how you perceive and respond to what is happening out there. Each of us creates the reality of our lives through selective acts of perception and interpretation. Given the same raw data of experience, people have very different responses because they interpret the experience through the filters of their personal history and unique mind body nature. If we wish to change our lives, we need to understand how we interpret the raw energy and information of the world and make a conscious choice to process things differently. Learning about our mind body constitution and choosing behaviors that are balancing to our nature are essential steps to enlivening our inherent vitality. Let's see how our nature can dramatically change the way we experience a situation. Given identical circumstances, an Earth, Fire, or Wind person will have differing interpretations of "reality." How do you think you would respond to the following situations?

Situation 1

You have reservations at a fine local restaurant but arrive twenty minutes late because of traffic that was heavier than expected. When you give your name to the maître d', he informs you that the restaurant has a policy of releasing a table if a patron is more than fifteen minutes late and yours is therefore no longer available. He politely apologizes and offers you the option of another table in about forty minutes.

EARTH RESPONSE. If Earth is the predominant element in your nature, you'll accept his offer, saunter over to the bar, and order some appetizers. If you feel irritated, you won't show it. If your spouse is less tolerant than you of this treatment, you'll try to pacify him or her and take the brunt of his or her irritation. When you are eventually given your table, you eat heartily, not only to assuage your hunger but also to relieve the empty emotional feeling in your gut. You become withdrawn during the evening, and after returning home promptly go to sleep.

FIRE RESPONSE. As a fiery being, your first response is irritation. You'll probably try to intimidate the maître d', and when you realize you are not getting your way, you may demand to speak with the owner of the restaurant. Your spouse's efforts to calm you down are met with irritation. With fire raging in your blood, you create only two possible outcomes of the confrontation: either you get a table or you storm out to another restaurant, vowing never to return. In either case, you are not likely to enjoy your meal that evening as you fume over the disrespectful treatment you received. You will also have some apologizing to do for bruising your spouse's feelings.

WIND RESPONSE. The Wind in your nature may well have been responsible for your being late in the first place. Trying to do too many things before getting ready for dinner, you hoped to make up for your tardiness by driving faster to the restaurant.

When you arrive late and are refused service, you feel embarrassed and apologetic. You try cajoling the maître d' into another table, using your most winning powers, but are careful to avoid any confrontation. Choosing to wait for the next table, you decide to take a walk and return at the anticipated hour. Passing a pay phone on the way out, you call another restaurant nearby to see if an earlier table is available. Throughout the experience you keep up a running conversation with your spouse about the thoughts going through your mind.

BALANCED RESPONSE. Components of each response would most likely enable you to achieve the best possible outcome while wasting the least amount of physical or emotional energy. Using your Earth energy, you could assume responsibility for your part in the problem without being overly ingratiating or patronizing. Your Fire component would request a firm commitment for the earliest available seating, and your Wind element would consider other options without making a disaster out of a minor mishap.

Situation 2
You are waiting at the airport for your cross-country flight when the airline representative announces that it has been delayed due to mechanical problems. They estimate it will take at least two hours before repairs can be made.

EARTH RESPONSE. You responsibly call your office and ask someone to contact the client who was supposed to meet you at your destination. You take the delay as an opportunity to eat an early lunch, and then enjoy the next couple of hours reading the novel you've been trying to get through for months.

FIRE RESPONSE. You become irritated at the delay and are not shy about expressing it. You demand that the agent find you a flight on another airline and threaten that arriving late for your meeting will have a serious impact on your business, for which the airline will pay.

WIND RESPONSE. You become anxious about missing your meeting and begin making urgent calls to your home office. Because you are only able to reach your assistant's voice mail, you frantically begin calling other airlines to see if you can get on an earlier plane. You learn that by accepting a flight that makes a stop, you can arrive three hours later than you were originally scheduled. You apologetically call your client to explain your predicament. She explains that she was trying to reach you to see if the meeting could be postponed until tomorrow.

BALANCED RESPONSE. The most effective responses are generally those that are not locked into a predictable pattern but draw on a variety of resources. In this case, accessing your Earth element and staying grounded ensures that you won't make the problem worse as a result of your reflexive reactions. The intensity of your Fire principle will add the appropriate level of urgency to the decisions that need to be made. Your Wind element keeps you from being complacent while you are considering your options.

Situation 3

Your sixteen-year-old son takes the car out for the first time without your direct supervision to go to a school party. You give him clear instructions to be home by 10:30 P.M., but by 11:00 he has not arrived home. Finally, at 11:45 the car pulls up, and your son casually saunters into the house.

EARTH RESPONSE. You are not prone to worry and assume your son is having a good time at the party. By eleven o'clock you are having trouble keeping your eyes open and decide to go to bed. When you hear your son enter the house, you ask him if he is all right. Upon learning that he is, you fall back to sleep. The next morning you talk to him about calling you if he is going to be late.

FIRE RESPONSE. You are fuming by the time he arrives home and chew him out about how irresponsible he is for coming home so late and failing to call. You take away his car keys and threaten not to return them until he has made amends. The next day, after you have cooled off, you feel bad about not controlling your anger with him, and within twenty-four hours he is back driving.

WIND RESPONSE. Your mind races with anxiety as you imagine the worst. By eleven o'clock you are calling your son's friends' houses to see if they have arrived home yet. By 11:30, you are literally pacing back and forth in front of the window searching for headlights. When he finally arrives, you don't know if you should hug him or spank him. Your first words are "How could you do this to me? Didn't you know how worried I would be?"

BALANCED RESPONSE. The primary goal of most parents would be to teach their son to behave more responsibly. Toward this end, a balanced approach would utilize all three forces. Drawing upon your Earth energy to maintain your calm is invariably helpful. Getting furiously angry or uncontrollably anxious is seldom an effective strategy for imparting wisdom. On the other hand, using your Fire energy to define a clear boundary and demonstrating that there a consistent, proportionate penalty to pay for infringement is teaching an important life lesson. Most parents would start to worry if their child was substantially late, and taking productive action by calling around is a good use of Wind energy.

There is not just one right way to deal with a stressful challenge. On the other hand, resorting to a predictable style that is governed by long-standing patterns limits your access to more effective strategies. The more balanced you are in body and mind, the more likely you will be able to react to stressful situations without losing your center. Responding from a state of balance tremendously enhances your likelihood of success while conserving valuable life energy.

Making Vital Energy Real

Observe the Mind Body Patterns around You

Just as understanding our own nature helps us to make choices in a more conscious way, identifying the inherent nature of those around us allows us to understand their behavior better. Understanding generates tolerance while enabling us to interact with people less stressfully and more successfully. See if you can characterize the major people in your life according to their predominant mind body principles. Notice how each person has a characteristic and often predictable way of reacting to challenges.

Person	Predominant Element(s)
Spouse or significant other	_____
Boss	_____
Mother	_____
Father	_____
Closest friend	_____
Children	_____

❁

I hope by now you have identified the forces that govern your mind and body and have recognized your patterns of response to stress that can lead you away from your vital center. You have made a diagnosis according to the timeless principles of the science of life—you have identified your primary nature and the tendencies that pull you off balance. You now know yourself at a new level.

The task at hand is how to use this knowledge to clear the obstacles that block access to your reservoir of energy, so you may recover the balance that brings vitality to body, mind, and soul. The next step in our journey is to digest the past, for only by digesting the past can we enter into the full potential of the present and envision a new future. It's time to release the toxic burdens that encumber your vitality.

Vital Energy Key #2

Clear Your Toxins,
Digest Your Past

The past is but the beginning of a beginning, and all that is
and has been is but the twilight of the dawn. —H. G. WELLS

I recently heard a story on the radio about a village in Pakistan
that had waited years for the government to install a sewer system.
Without one, the residents disposed of their refuse by dumping
buckets of waste into the alley. As a result, their infant mortality
rate was one of the highest in the world, with their children dying
from a host of infectious illnesses. Finally, the villagers decided
they could no longer wait for the government to fulfill its promise
and decided to build the disposal system on their own. Within a
year, the health of the community was transformed. Not only
were the vast majority of babies living to see their first birthday,
but crime fell, the economy improved, and new cooperative projects were initiated with unprecedented enthusiasm.

This story illustrates a basic principle of Ayurveda—if we retain substances that are meant to be eliminated, the accumulation of toxicity depletes our life force. If we eliminate toxic congestion, our creativity, enthusiasm, and well being flourish. This is as true for our physical and mental health as it is for our environment. We carry the past in our environment, bodies, hearts, and minds, and when the burden becomes too heavy, we lose the ability to prosper in the present. Therefore, identifying, healing, and releasing unprocessed experiences are essential for restoring our natural vitality.

Novelist Tom Robbins wrote that there are really only two mantras in life: "yum" and "yuck." Anything we ingest can have either a nourishing or toxic effect on our minds and bodies, depending upon what it is, how much we are exposed to, and our ability to metabolize the energy and information that it contains. Too little or too much of the vital gas oxygen is harmful to health. Too little or too much food can make us unhappy and unwell. A lack of love can certainly make us sick, as can too much, as when an overprotective mother denies her children the freedom to make their own choices.

Even a nourishing substance may have a toxic effect if we are not able to fully digest and absorb it. If you are lacking lactase, the enzyme necessary to digest milk sugar, a cup of hot cocoa may cause bloating and cramping. If you have recently disentangled yourself from an abusive relationship, even a friendly overture from someone attracted to you may feel invasive. A lecture at your local college on the latest theory of creation may sound fascinating, but if the speaker's vocabulary confuses rather than illuminates, you may be left with mental indigestion rather than satisfying food for thought.

Everything in the natural world has potential value. There is a rich mythology surrounding Jivaka, a famous Ayurvedic physician at the time of Buddha. While Jivaka was still a medical student, his teacher sent his class to the countryside to retrieve items that were devoid of any medicinal value. Each of the students returned with many different things—weeds, rocks, lizards—which they considered medically valueless. After a day of searching, Jivaka returned empty-handed, stating that he could not find a single natural item that did not have potential healing value. Every mineral, plant, and animal was therapeutic in the right context. Gazing at the clouds, listening to the brook, or experiencing the caress of a summer breeze had a possible healing effect on body and mind.

Jivaka might have more difficulty saying the same thing about the world today. Over the past hundred years we have introduced millions of new synthetic chemicals into our environment which, although they may provide some advantage in a very localized domain, have a toxic effect on our mental or physical well being in minute concentrations. As we'll explore during this chapter, if we wish to restore our vitality, we need to honestly evaluate our collective tolerance for pollution at every level of our lives and consciously choose to eliminate toxicity from our air, water, and earth, as well as from our bodies, emotions, and beliefs.

Explore the Layers of Your Life

We are composed of interwoven layers of life, each of which must be clear for us to feel vital and enthusiastic. Our intentions and desires arise from the deepest level of our being and are then expressed through our beliefs, emotions, and physical body. Our aspirations are most readily fulfilled when vital energy flows effortlessly through the layers of our lives. Unfortunately, we can accumulate toxins in our environment, body, emotions, and mind. Although our soul is beyond the realm of imbalance and disease, its light can be overshadowed by the encumbrances we carry. Adi Shankara, a great Vedic sage around A.D. 500, described human life as composed of layers. When each layer is free from toxicity, we experience life as magical and enchanting. When there are blockages to the free flow of vital energy, we feel alienated and depleted.

Our first layer, known as the *bliss sheath*, contains our deepest desires in embryonic form. In the right season, seeds of desire sprout, giving rise to our aspirations and longings. They form our core impulses for achieving fulfillment in our relationships and work. The hopes we carry for meeting our soul mate, the goals we have for achieving fame and fortune, and our longing for understanding the deeper meaning of life have their roots in the bliss sheath. At different stages of our lives, different desires arise. As children we long for dolls and bicycles. As teenagers we drool over a medley of animate and inanimate objects of infatuation, from cars to rock stars. We want to look good at this stage and usually take our health for granted. As young adults we feel the hunger for exciting jobs, attractive lovers, and symbols of material success. Later many of us feel the desire for a family and a home in which to raise it. Under the strain of these responsibilities many people feel some waning of their vitality; they feel the desire for the restoration of energy they need to enjoy life. If our basic personal longings are fulfilled, we enter a stage when our desire to serve our local and global communities blossoms. Finally, sooner or later, most people become aware of a deeper longing in their souls to understand and experience a connection with something that transcends their individuality and community—call it nature, spirit, or God. This first layer holds all these seeds that eventually germinate into the intentions and desires of our lives. Having access to our source of vital energy is the only way to ensure that our deepest desires will be realized.

The next layer is the *idea sheath*. It is here that we carry the thoughts and beliefs we hold to be true in our lives. What we believe about ourselves and those around us resonates in this layer. We place ourselves at the center of the universe and believe that our view of the world is true and accurate. We form our layer of ideas by listening to the conversations around us. The perspectives of our families, community, country, and world shape our view of reality. We look at "truths" prevailing on the planet in earlier eras and can only imagine what it must have been like to believe the sun revolved around the earth or that evil spirits caused infectious diseases. People living during the time of the Roman Empire, the Renaissance, or the dawn of the Industrial Revolution believed in their reality as completely as we believe in ours. There is little doubt that future generations will look back at our age and wonder how we could have possibly thought the things we do.

We are witnessing a shift in our personal and collective idea layer. Building upon the insights of the great scientists of the twentieth century, we are seeing tangible changes in our daily lives. We have entered the Age of Information, and each one of us is affected by the recognition that information is subtler and more powerful than matter. Fax machines, cellular phones, digital video equipment, laptop computers, and satellite television are testaments to the advent of this new age. In prior ages, the wealthiest people and wealthiest countries had the most stuff—gold, jewels, oil reserves. Today wealth is measured in terms of the ability to access and use information and energy. We now recognize that everything that appears to be solid and material is merely a form of energy and information. Understanding this at the level of our idea layer is essential for us to access our inner reservoir of vital energy. If we don't know it exists, we won't find it.

The next layer beyond our beliefs is the *emotional sheath*, the domain of our feelings. The more love and appreciation we've experienced in our lives, the healthier and more vital this layer is for us. If you were raised believing you deserved love just for being alive, your emotional layer is probably relatively healthy. You expect to be appreciated and respected in your relationships and will not tolerate people who treat you otherwise. If, on the other hand, your caregivers were immersed in their own emotional turmoil, you probably received lots of mixed messages about how and who you needed to be in order to deserve love. As a consequence, your relationships tend to be turbulent and there always seems to be something missing. Unfortunately, this is the experience of many people I see. Identifying and releasing inappropriate emotional messages and replacing them with honoring, nurturing ones is essential to mental and physical vitality.

Next we enter into our *physical sheath*, composed of energy and matter. When our physical bodies effortlessly exchange energy and information with our environment, we experience vitality, immunity, and vigor. When we accumulate toxicity in the body, we require increasing amounts of energy to perform the same function and experience exhaustion and depletion. The body is the end product of our experiences in life. An ancient Ayurvedic expression suggests that you can know your past experiences by looking at your body now, and can predict the quality of your body in the future by examining your experiences now. To create a healthy body, we need to imbibe life-supporting impulses while incinerating retained toxicity from the past.

Let's look further at these different layers of life and see how we can eliminate the obstacles to our unrestricted vitality.

Making Vital Energy Real

Navigate Your Layers

Consider the current health of each layer of your life. What is working and what needs some attention? Spend a few minutes honestly assessing the areas where you are wealthy and those where you are needy. Respond to each question below and reflect on your unfiltered responses. Then ask yourself: what small step can I take today to enhance my quality of living?

1. My layer of deepest desires. What do I really want . . .
In my relationships?

_____

_____

_____

In my work?

_____

_____

_____

In my spiritual life?

_____

_____

_____

2. My layer of beliefs

_____

_____

_____

What beliefs do I hold about myself and the world that are useful and empowering?

_____
_____
_____

What beliefs do I hold about myself and the world that are unproductive and disempowering?

_____
_____
_____

3. My layer of emotions
What is working in my emotional life?

_____
_____
_____

What needs work in my emotional life?

_____
_____
_____

4. My physical layer

_____
_____
_____

In what ways am I attentive and nurturing to the needs of my body?

_____
_____
_____

In what ways am I inattentive or neglectful to the needs of my body?

_____
_____
_____

Embrace Your Environment

We are becoming increasingly aware of the interconnectedness of all beings on this planet. The same technology that threatens our ecology alerts us that our survival depends upon our species acting as responsible stewards for our world. According to Ayurveda, the environment is an extension of our physical body. When I first heard this, I thought it was an interesting metaphor, but the more I explored the idea, the more I realized it was true. Our bodies and our environments are in constant and dynamic exchange with one another. In his fascinating book *The Seven Mysteries of Life*, Guy Murchie calculates that twenty thousand times each day we breathe in and breathe out ten billion trillion (10^{22}) atoms. Further calculations lead to the amazing finding that we claim ownership in our body of a quadrillion (10^{15}) atoms that have been in someone else's body within the past few weeks. Perhaps even more mind-boggling is the math that demonstrates that at any moment, each of us has at least a million atoms in our body that were once in the body of every person who has ever lived, from Moses to Madonna, Isaac Newton to Newt Gingrich.

The average human body has about ten trillion quadrillion (10^{28}) atoms at any one time. Radioisotope studies show that about 98 percent of these physical building blocks are completely exchanged within one year, and within five years the last jealously held atom in a nerve cell or tendon is replaced. It is scientifically accurate to say that at the atomic level we trade in our old body for a new model about fifteen times during our lifetime. As living beings, we are continuously recycling our elements with the elements of our environment. We transform the energy and information of food, water, and air into the energy and information of our bodies, while simultaneously returning molecular bits and pieces of our bodies back to the environment. The superficial layer of our skin, the largest organ of the body, is completely shed and replaced within about one month. The lining of our stomach is swapped every week, and our liver turns over about nine times a year. You may identify closely with your body, but the truth of the matter is that the molecules that compose your body are only on temporary loan to you from the environmental library.

If as a society we collectively grasped the intimacy we share with our environment, we would dramatically change the way we treat the spaceship upon which we are traveling. Most people would not consciously defecate in their living room or throw out their garbage in their backyard, yet the toxicity we deposit in our environment is every bit as irrational and harmful. In a recent edition of the textbook *Environmental Medicine*, Drs. Stuart M. Brooks, Lynette Benson, and Michael Gochfeld present this startling picture of our current environmental plight.

> At present there are at least 26 groups of chemicals known to be human carcinogens, over 600 known rodent carcinogens, over 2000 known teratogens [inducers of birth defects], and more than 50,000 chemicals or chemical compounds with no scientific study of toxicity. Over 1400 active ingredients are formulated into more than 45,000 pesticide products. More than 6 billion tons of toxic waste with diverse chemical compositions are produced each year. Of the 5 to 6 million chemicals with a known molecular structure, 60,000 of which are currently in use in agricultural, manufacturing, or medical applications, only about 1% have been tested for toxicity. The problem of assessing toxicity is compounded by the fact that approximately 6000 new chemicals are synthesized each week.

Light One Candle: Eliminate One Toxin at a Time

What can we do about the toxicity in our environment? The first step is to become aware of our collective tolerance for chemicals in our air, water, soil, and food. Every time I drive my gas-guzzling car, refuse to buy a tomato that has a single mark on it, throw away a plastic cup after a single drink, or spray insect repellent in my kitchen to eradicate ants that have arrived for a midnight snack, I am contributing to the toxicity in my environment. Tomorrow morning, pay attention to the number of synthetic substances you encounter even before you leave the house. You are exposed to chemicals in your soap, shampoo, hair conditioner, hair spray, deodorant, toothpaste, mouthwash, makeup, nail polish, shoe polish, dishwashing liquid, and laundry detergent. Although you may be operating under the assumption that the preservatives, dyes, and fragrances in these products have been proven safe, even the FDA's own scientists have recently issued concerns about the potential risks of chemicals in common household commodities.

A major problem with environmental pollution is that most of the time it is invisible. Benzene from automobile exhausts, carbon monoxide from furnaces, lead in the drinking water, and chloroform from incinerators do not announce their presence with flashing lights or clanging bells. The tens of thousands of chemicals that pervade our air, water, and soil are, for the most part, silent, invisible toxins. Only rarely does an acute disaster, such as the Bhopal pesticide plant catastrophe that killed over two thousand people or the Chernobyl nuclear accident that exposed over half the world's population to radioactive contamination, grab the headlines.

Unfortunately, we tolerate the daily release of industrial waste into our water supply, low-level radioactivity into our air, and pesticides into our soil with barely a whimper. The Environmental Protection Agency (EPA) and other local and state organizations are watching out for us, but environmental policy derives from a political process, and there are many highly invested stakeholders whose interests may not best serve the public. An industry that makes or uses a potentially toxic substance will put the burden of proof on those who are apprehensive about its harm, whereas a concerned citizen wants the chemical to be withheld until it is clearly proven to be safe.

As our collective concern for the environment has risen over the past twenty-five years, we have seen some signs of hope. According to the EPA, we can document a decrease in many common air pollutants, toxic pesticides, lead, and ozone-depleting chemicals. Unfortunately, 62 million Americans still live in metropolitan areas that fail to meet air quality standards, greenhouse gases have risen worldwide, and 40 percent of our rivers and lakes are not clean enough to meet basic fishing and swimming standards. Although recycling of paper, plastic, and glass has tripled since 1970, we have increased solid waste production to 209 million tons per day, which is more than four pounds per American, up by a third since twenty-five years ago.

Considering the magnitude of the problem, mustering the energy to do something about it may seem pointless. However, each of us needs to take greater responsibility for our personal contribution to toxicity in the environment—our extended body. On an individual basis, we each can choose to make a difference, no matter how small it may seem. Rather than assuming that the problem is too big for one person to influence, take a small step in the direction of contributing to the solution by changing some aspect of your behavior. When a critical mass of people becomes conscious of how our daily choices contribute to our collective experience, we will see a transformation in the world. Our personal and collective vitality depends upon it.

Making Vital Energy Real

Clean Your Space
1. Whenever possible, walk, jog, ride your bicycle, or Rollerblade rather than automatically using your fossil-fuel–consuming vehicle for short trips.
2. Recycle all cans, plastic containers, and paper products, and always favor items that use minimal packaging.
3. Get in the habit of carrying reusable bags and containers rather than relying on disposables. The best answer to "paper or plastic?" is neither.
4. Never discharge toxic waste materials into the water supply or onto the ground. This includes automobile fluids, paint thinners, cleaning supplies, or other industrial chemicals. Find recycling centers in your community that accept and appropriately dispose of, or recycle, industrial waste.
5. Minimize your use of synthetic pesticides, herbicides, and fertilizers on your lawn and garden. Use nontoxic alternatives for your household cleaning needs.
6. Align your financial resources with your beliefs. Spend a few more cents on organic fruits, vegetables, and dairy products that avoid pesticides and synthetic fertilizers.

7. Consider a political candidate's environmental views when voting. Think long-term when balancing economic and environmental issues.

Clear Your Senses

Jim couldn't figure out what was wrong with him. As a successful floor trader at the New York Stock Exchange, he had been living on the energy of raw capitalism for the past five years. Although his work was intense, he prided himself on his ability to leave the tumult behind when he left the building. But lately, he was having increasing difficulty sleeping at night and had to drag himself out of bed in the morning.

When he came to see me about his ongoing fatigue, I learned that other than this visit to San Diego, he had not been outside New York City for at least three years. He lived within a mile of Wall Street and spent his life focused entirely on his work. His senses were overloaded with the sounds, sensations, sights, and smells of an intense city.

Although he was expecting prescriptions for nutritional substances to "give me more energy," I made only two recommendations: Practice meditation on a daily basis, and get out of the city at least twice a month. When he called me several weeks later, he sounded like a different person. His enthusiasm for life had returned, and he had rediscovered the value of feeding his senses with simpler, natural experiences.

Sound

We ingest the world through our digestive tract, our breathing passages, and our five senses. If the sounds, sensations, sights, smells, and tastes are nourishing to body, mind, and soul, we are more likely to transform the energy of our environment into vital energy. A sensory environment that is harsh and abrasive offends our sensibilities, and we experience rawness and fatigue. Studies looking at pregnancy outcomes have shown that mothers living close to a noisy airport are more likely to have small babies. Even young children who live in noisy inner-city neighborhoods are more likely to have high blood pressure than their suburban counterparts.

Noise pollution erodes everyone's quality of life and is one of the most common complaints of people working and living in high-density urban buildings. If you are feeling chronically fatigued, pay attention to the sounds that surround you. On a regular basis, go to places where the only sounds you hear are sounds of nature—chirping crickets, warbling birds, flowing streams. Change your daily sensory environment to provide nourishing, rather than toxic, inputs. Play uplifting music or the sounds of nature in your work and home surroundings. If you cannot spend more of your time in nature, bring nature into your living spaces.

You can fine-tune your "sound therapy" based on your mind body type. Earth types generally feel invigorated by music with a more driving beat and melody. Rock and roll, rap, drumming, spirited world music, and passionate classical pieces can help get the Earth moving. Fire types get balanced with cooler, sweeter sounds. Cool jazz, flute music, and Mozart can soothe the ferocious impulses of a potent Fire man or woman. The calming sounds of nature—falling rain, ocean waves, or bubbling streams—can also cool excessive heat. If Wind is your dominant energy, listen to sounds that are warm and grounding. Bach cello partitas, calming New Age pieces, and Gregorian chants can provide the balancing vibrations needed to quell the turbulence. Use these basic principles as guidelines, but listen to your body while you are listening to the sounds around you and choose the tones and tunes that feel good to you.

Touch

Our skin is the boundary between the environment and ourselves. The largest organ in the body, our skin is an important source of natural healing and rejuvenating chemicals. The value of therapeutic touch is regaining importance as study after study demonstrates its value in reducing stress and enhancing immunity. Wonderful, professional massages are not the only way to benefit from therapeutic touch. Try this simple self-massage on a daily basis, and you will promptly notice an improvement in your state of well being.

FULL BODY MASSAGE. Begin by massaging a tablespoon of warm oil onto your scalp with small circular strokes, as if shampooing. Move to the face and ears, massaging more gently. Gentle massage of the temples and backs of the ears is especially good for settling the Wind element.

Massage a small amount of oil onto the neck, front and back, and then the shoulders. Vigorously massage the arms, using a circular motion at the shoulders and elbows, and long back-and-forth motions on the upper arms and forearms. Using large, gentle circular motions, massage the chest, stomach, and lower abdomen. A straight up-and-down motion can be used over the breastbone.

After applying a bit of oil to both hands, gently reach around to massage the back and spine as best you can. Use an up-and-down motion. As with the arms, vigorously massage the legs with a circular motion at the ankles and knees, straight back-and-forth on the long parts. Use whatever oil remains to vigorously massage the feet. Pay extra attention to your toes.

Earth types benefit from more vigorous body work that enlivens the circulation. You can even perform the self-massage with a dry cotton or linen glove to maximize its stimulating effect. Fire types do best with deep tissue massage that encourages release of muscle tension and pressure. Wind people generally need gentler therapeutic touch and should be careful to stay warm during any massage.

Sight

Pay attention to the visual stimuli in your environment. Whenever possible, choose to allow nourishing rather than toxic images into your awareness. Watching movies or television shows that are continuously laced with violence create nearly the same experience of stress as if you were directly involved in the traumatic conflicts. Regularly seek out the sights of a natural environment and strive to surround yourself with images that are elevating to your spirit.

If you are earthy by nature, enlivening visual stimuli can help you tap into your energy source. Brighter colors and bolder patterns in your clothing and environment can lighten you up. Fiery types benefit from a more cooling visual environment. Taking walks by natural bodies of water and in verdant parks can keep you from overheating. Cooler blues and greens in your home and work environments can have a balancing effect. Wind spirits need visual grounding, which can be provided through earth tones and lush nature scenes.

Smell

Olfaction is our most primitive sense and is intimately connected to our memory and feelings. For most of our animal forerunners, the bulk of the brain is dedicated to the processing of olfactory information obtained from the environment. Creatures from wombats to wolves are continuously sniffing the ground and air for clues about the world. The sense of smell is intimately interwoven with memory and emotion in the limbic lobe of the brain and is used by most mammals and reptiles to identify food, danger, and possible reproductive mates. As a neurology resident I learned the four "F's" of the limbic system, which were feeding, fighting, fleeing, and the four-letter word for the act of reproduction. In early days of our evolutionary journey, smell was the primary sense that activated these basic components of survival. Although as *Homo sapiens* we usually do not pay much conscious attention to the sense of smell, we still inhale tremendous amounts of olfactory information about the world, triggering memories and emotions. A whiff of perfume can flood your mind with recollections and feelings of an ancient love affair. The smell of a puppy's breath can access childhood memories that have been latent for decades. Scientific studies demonstrate that smells can calm or invigorate.

Experiment with natural scents and aromas, and surround yourself with those that enhance your well being.

Different scents can have specific effects to balance overactive mind body energies. Light, stimulating smells can invigorate congested Earth types. Cooling, refreshing aromas are beneficial for Fire types, while warm, grounding smells work best to calm turbulent Wind constitutions. Specific suggestions for balancing fragrances are listed below, but as is true for all the senses, give primary attention to the feedback you receive from your body. The essential questions to be asked are "Do I like this aroma?" and "How does it make me feel?"

Aromas to Invigorate	Aromas to Cool	Aromas to Calm
Lemon	Jasmine	Lavender
Orange	Mint	Vanilla
Clove	Lime	Sandalwood
Cinnamon	Rose	Neroli

Making Vital Energy Real

Nourish Your Senses

Tune in to your senses. Pay attention to the sounds, sensations, sights, and smells in your environment. To the extent possible, reduce those sensory inputs that are toxic and augment those that are nourishing. Spend today surrounding yourself with wonderful sounds, sights, sensations, and smells. Become aware of the influence of your sensory world on your sense of vitality.

Purify Your Body: What Is Your Toxin Load?

Identifying, avoiding, and neutralizing toxins from our bodies are key to freeing up vital energy, for our bodies are the end products of our experiences in life. To recapture vitality, we need to eliminate accumulated toxins and minimize our exposure to situations and circumstances that have a toxic influence.

Take this simple toxicity quiz, answering each question as honestly as possible.

Toxicity Survey	Does not apply at all	Applies to some extent	Applies to a great extent
1. At least five days per week I consume sources of animal fat.	1	3	5
2. I regularly smoke cigarettes.	1	3	5
3. I drink alcoholic beverages on a regular basis.	1	3	5
4. I regularly use non-prescription mind-altering drugs.	1	3	5
5. I live in a city that has noticeable air pollution.	1	3	5
6. I regularly consume junk foods.	1	3	5
7. I experience considerable stress at work.	1	3	5
8. I am often depressed.	1	3	5
9. I regularly find myself in emotionally abusive relationships.	1	3	5
10. I consume caffeine-containing beverages on a regular basis.	1	3	5

Total Toxicity Score _____

Your body is the stage upon which your mind plays out its dramas. It can be a battlefield or a playground, depending on your life's script. If you are feeling mentally and physically depleted, it is because accumulated toxicity has exceeded your capacity to metabolize and discharge it. In modern scientific terms, we might say that you have accumulated an oxidative debt with more free radical production than you have the ability to neutralize, resulting in toxic damage to your cells and biochemicals. From whatever perspective we approach it, the conclusion is clear—if we wish to live a life filled with vitality, we need to treat our bodies with reverence. This means assessing every aspect of our daily choices and opting for those that are life supporting rather than life damaging.

Tally up your score from the toxicity questionnaire. If you scored fewer than 20 points, you are living a relatively pure life and probably look and feel younger than your chronological age. If your score falls between 20 and 35 points, you can definitely improve your vitality by paying attention to and reducing your regular exposure to experiences that do not offer nourishment. Above 35 points, you have some serious life-damaging habits to break. The good news is that if you dedicate yourself to reducing your exposure to toxins, you will see a rapid improvement in your vital energy level.

Life is amazingly forgiving up to a point, after which our adaptive mechanisms become overloaded and the forces of entropy begin to overpower the orderly forces of living systems. Make the changes in your lifestyle before you get to a point where recovering your balance is very difficult. You will experience immediate as well as long-term benefits.

The Oxygen Paradox

We are raised in a sea of oxygen; we are completely dependent upon this vital gas for our myriad biological activities. Within ten seconds of oxygen deprivation our brain shuts down; after ten minutes irreversible damage occurs. Although oxygen is an exceedingly rare commodity in the grander universe, it constitutes one in five atoms in the earth's atmosphere and one in four atoms in our bodies. Oxygen is ultimately responsible for both life and death, for oxygen's presence in almost every biochemical reaction leads to the formation of free radicals that underlie most, if not all, illnesses.

Free radicals are highly unstable, potentially destructive molecules that react with the nearest chemical as soon as they are created. These nasty beasts go by a number of different names—singlet oxygen, hydrogen peroxide, hydroxy radical—but they all have one thing in common: they have an intense appetite for electrons. A free radical's raging atomic hunger leads to almost indiscriminate bonding with the nearest molecule: proteins, carbohydrates, fats, DNA molecules—free radicals are not particular. Accumulated insults as a result of these reactions underlie most human illnesses, from arthritis to Alzheimer's disease, cancer to coronary heart disease. In essence, biological aging is the accumulation of oxidative damage due to free radicals.

As living beings on planet earth, we cannot avoid free radical molecules. We therefore have developed a highly sophisticated system to neutralize them as soon as possible after they have formed. Known as our antioxidant defenses, some components of this system serve as sacrificial lambs offered to the free radical monsters while others have evolved the ability to rapidly neutralize the destructive creatures before they cause any damage. Inactivating enzymes such as superoxide dismutase (SOD) and glutathione peroxidase are not commonly known by the general public, but the antioxidant vitamins C, E, A, and beta-carotene have been in the public consciousness for years. We are learning that a vast variety of plant-derived chemicals are also potent free radical quenchers. These phytochemicals (*phyto* means plant) will be explored in greater detail in the next chapter, but for now, it is helpful to recognize that there are many compounds in fruits, vegetables, and whole grains that provide protection from marauding oxygen molecules.

In addition to ensuring that our diet is rich in antioxidant nutrients, what more can we do to counteract the ravages of free radicals? The answer is simple: we can reduce the toxic influences that fuel the production of free radicals. This means reducing our exposure to toxic air, food, substances, and emotions. Whenever we activate our stress response, the revving up of our physiology generates free radicals. The hormones released under stress—adrenaline and cortisol—trigger chemical cascades that gulp oxygen and create a flurry of oxidizing by-products. The more often we activate a stress response, the more free radicals are formed.

The toxins we consume on a daily basis also contribute to our free radical load. Cigarette smoke and alcohol create oxidative stress, which over time predisposes our cells to cancer and degenerative disorders. Barbecued and smoked meats, processed foods, and aged cheeses all contribute to free radical production. Many environmental chemicals, chemotherapy drugs, and radiation, including sunlight, activate free radicals and can eventually cause biochemical and cellular disruption.

Eliminating Toxic Behaviors

Most people know that smoking cigarettes, excessive alcohol intake, recreational drugs, overeating, and too much red meat are destructive and depleting of vitality. The quintessential question is how can you change your undesirable behaviors? There are really only two reasons to do things differently from the way you usually do: first, you want to avoid pain, or second, you anticipate greater pleasure. To eliminate a behavior such as cigarette smoking, you need to experience the direct negative effect of the habit and find an alternative approach that satisfies the need smoking has been fulfilling. The most effective way to experience the harmful effects of a behavior is to bring your full awareness into the process. Try this exercise:

> When you are about to smoke your next cigarette, stop whatever else you are doing and find a quiet place, free from distractions. Do not smoke while you are working, driving, talking on the phone, or engaged in conversation. Close your eyes and take a few slow deep breaths. Scan your body and see if you can identify where in your body you are experiencing the craving for the cigarette. Simply observe the sensation without judgment or resistance, allowing any tension in that area of your body to dissipate with each exhalation of your breath.
>
> When you are ready, reach for your pack of cigarettes with total awareness. Witness yourself taking a cigarette from the pack, placing it in your mouth, and lighting the

match. With undivided attention experience all the sensations associated with your first inhalation. Feel the sensations in your mouth, throat, and lungs as you inhale the smoke. Experience the smells and tastes with your eyes closed. Once per minute repeat the process until your desire has been satiated; then put out the cigarette.

This same procedure can be used with any addictive behavior. If you have a chocolate addiction, eat a piece of chocolate with total awareness. If you binge on junk foods, eat your Cheese Puffs or Fritos with your full attention. Most people who practice this technique find that their urge to indulge is promptly satiated without having to binge. If you have the clear intention to relinquish your attachment and innocently listen to your body's response to the experience, you will find the habit loosening its hold on your mind and body.

Making Vital Energy Real

Banish Toxicity from Your Life

1. Eliminate tobacco from your life today. To satisfy your oral needs, try sucking on a cinnamon stick or a clove bud.
2. Reduce your alcohol consumption. If you have lost control over your drinking, seek professional help or join your local Alcoholics Anonymous group.
3. Eliminate the use of all nonessential drugs. Try natural alternatives to the chronic use of sleeping medications, anxiety drugs, or chronic pain relievers.
4. Reduce your intake of barbecued, smoked, and aged meats and cheeses.
5. Use sunblock whenever you are outside. Skin cancer is a high price to pay for skin that is a few shades darker.
6. Increase your intake of foods rich in antioxidant vitamins. Fresh fruits, vegetables, and whole grains are the richest sources.
7. Manage your stress. Take time each day to meditate.

Simplify and Detoxify

When our physiology is young and strong, we carry a sense of invincibility. Each day I see people in consultation who have lived intensely, without much regard for the consequences of their choices. Then at a time later in their lives, their bodies demonstrate the effects of the previous choices. I recently spent time with a man who exemplifies this process.

Stan was forty-seven years old going on seventy. He had been regulating his moods with drugs since his high school days. As an adult, he was able to build a successful manufacturing business that provided him with the resources to buy higher quality cocaine and alcohol. When his stomach began to swell, he initially assumed his rich diet was giving him middle-age spread, but when his girth continued to expand, he sought medical attention. After a series of tests, it was determined that he had cirrhosis of the liver due to a combination of drinking and a past viral hepatitis infection. This was the alarm that finally woke Stan up to pay attention to his body.

In Western medicine, the term *detoxification* is usually applied to withdrawal from addictive drug or alcohol use. We recognize that removing a person from a toxic behavior allows him or her to reestablish a healthier boundary between the inner need and the substance that only temporarily satisfies the need. As the substance—be it tobacco, alcohol, or a drug—is withdrawn, people experience distress until their internal pharmacy reestablishes equilibrium. Once the toxic influence is removed, healing can begin and higher levels of comfort and well being can be accessed.

We can expand this approach to less obvious sources of toxicity. If we are used to intense sensory stimulation with blaring music, powerful images, and concentrated sensations, withdrawal from these impressions may initially generate uncomfortable feelings. People accustomed to eating while watching television or always having the news on while at work may feel uneasy when they first change their behavior. People dependent upon their cups of coffee, Diet Cokes, or double cheeseburgers may not experience full-blown withdrawal symptoms if they go without for a few days, but they do feel unsettled and often have intrusive thoughts about the substance they have become used to. Human beings are capable of becoming hooked on almost anything— food, sex, power, relationships, thrills—and withdrawal from the object of attachment, whatever it is, manifests itself with similar sensations.

This does not mean that in order to be vital we need to live a life free from intense experiences. On the contrary, the more balanced we are in mind and body, the more we are able to ardently enjoy the sensory world. The difference is in our level of attachment to the experience. If we need a powerful stimulus just to feel alive, we are surrendering our vitality to something outside ourselves and will always feel vulnerable. If we are fulfilled and connected to the deepest levels of our nature, we are able to extract the nourishment from every experience that comes our way.

If you have a predominance of Earth in your nature, seek out experiences that are vitally dynamic. Take a vigorous hike through the woods, ride your bike in the park, or swim in the lake. Imbibe the life force with enthusiasm to enliven your circulation. If you are a fiery type, focus on sensory nourishment that brings you into the present moment. Walk along the shoreline at sunset, go scuba diving, or make love for hours. Take some time to experience the timeless moments of life. If your windy nature keeps you perpetually on the brink of turbulence, choose nourishing experiences that create safety for you. Seek out natural hot springs, get warm massages, and make yourself delicious vegetable soups. Whatever intrinsic mind body constitution you express, use the elements of nature to nourish and balance your body, mind, and soul.

Taking time to withdraw our senses from the world attunes and enlivens our ability to enjoy. If you haven't eaten for a while, food tastes more delicious. If you haven't had physical intimacy for a time, sex is more sumptuous. With every sense, taking the opportunity to withdraw allows for more fulfilling sensory experiences. I encourage you to take detoxification retreats on a regular basis. Tuning in to the subtler sensory impulses of nature—birds singing, streams flowing, the warmth of the sun—will balance and heal you.

Making Vital Energy Real

Purifying Action Steps

There are a number of approaches that can help you release accumulated toxins. Take an inward stroke for one or several days to allow your body to detoxify from the pressure and stresses of your daily life. I do not recommend that you try these approaches when you are in the middle of a demanding time. Wait until, or create, a break that allows you to purify and nourish yourself.

* Follow a liquefied diet. Try it a couple times per month if you have a predominance of Earth, a few times a year if you have a predominance of Fire, and only rarely if Wind is your predominant element. Take in only freshly squeezed fruit and vegetable juices throughout the day. Try fruit juices in the morning, fruit and vegetable mixtures during the middle part of the day, and primarily vegetable juices in the evening. Experiment with carrots, apples, beets, grapes, spinach, and citrus fruits. Sip gingerroot tea prepared by adding one teaspoon of freshly grated ginger to one pint of hot water.
* If a liquefied diet seems too extreme for you, follow a simplified diet. Eat only fresh fruits, vegetables, rice, and easily digestible legumes such as mung beans or red lentils. Consume fresh fruits in the morning, vegetables and rice during the day, and soup at night. Avoid milk, meat, eggs, cheese, and refined carbohydrates.
* Spend time in silence. Turn off your phones, radios, and television and simply witness your thoughts throughout the day. Practice yoga and meditation and read books that are elevating to the human spirit. Observe the thought activity in your mind without judgment and listen to the silence that is there beneath the turbulence.
* Gently nurture your body and mind through your senses. Get a massage, listen to soothing music, and diffuse purifying aromas in your environment—sandalwood, clary sage, jasmine, citrus. Go to a beautiful environment and connect with nature. Take off your shoes and wiggle your toes in the earth. Walk along a natural body of water and feel its soothing influ-

ence. Luxuriate in the warmth of the sun. Visit a botanical garden and take slow deep breaths, inhaling the oxygen-rich breath of plants and trees. Lie on your back and gaze up into the sky, watching the clouds float by.

- Spend the day journaling. Ask yourself the question "Why am I here?" and see what answers arise in your awareness. Ask yourself "What hurts, frustrations, and resentments am I carrying in my heart, and what I can do to release them?" Allow your inner mind to respond without attempting to control or filter.

A Word on Chronic Fatigue Syndrome

Not having enough energy is one of the most common reasons people seek medical attention. If you complain to your doctor that you are feeling exhausted a lot of the time, he or she will probably order a series of tests to rule out treatable causes for your fatigue. You will most likely have your blood tested for anemia, an underactive thyroid, AIDS, diabetes, and kidney and liver diseases. Depending on your age, you may go through a series of tests to be certain that you do not have a malignancy. Once you have completed all your studies, the chances are good that no specific medical condition will be diagnosed to account for your fatigue.

At this point your doctor will likely be at a loss to explain your lack of vitality and may suggest you try an antidepressant medication. If you are among the small percentage of people who are extremely tired all of the time, the term *chronic fatigue syndrome* (CFS) may be suggested. When unrelenting tiredness is associated with chronic pain, depression, and immune weakness, we now apply the label chronic fatigue syndrome. Although the label *CFS* has been around only since 1987, healing systems for millennia have recognized that people can be overwhelmed by feelings of persistent mental and physical depletion. A focus on Epstein-Barr virus as a cause for CFS was popular in the 1980s, but most researchers now believe that alterations in viral measurements reflect a mild immune system imbalance rather than a specific viral infection accounting for the fatigue.

Applying the diagnosis of CFS gives the impression that modern medicine understands this condition, but unfortunately this is not the case. The label CFS is merely a description of different symptoms that are sometimes expressed together. Medicine knows neither the cause nor the treatment for the condition. People who receive this diagnosis sometimes mistakenly believe they have a well-characterized disease and anticipate medical science will provide a cure.

Although it may be frustrating to learn that the diagnosis of CFS is little more than a description of the problem, the lack of definition can be an opportunity for healing. I believe it is much more accurate to view this condition as an exaggerated state of mind body imbalance than as a specific disease. From a holistic perspective the lack of energy experienced by people with CFS represents a lack of integration among body, mind, and soul. The treatment should require the identification and removal of the obstacles that are inhibiting the flow of vital energy. Regardless of where you are on the spectrum of vitality, reconnecting with your inner source of energy is essential to invigorate your life. To accomplish this, you must eliminate toxicity from your life.

Remove the Obstacles to Vital Energy

All living beings face a similar challenge. Whether you are an amoeba or *Homo sapiens*, you need to consume energy and information from your environment to survive and thrive. Most of the time, the substances that are consumed come with biochemical accessories that may not be nourishing and therefore need to be disposed of. The ability to efficiently ingest, digest, and eliminate determines the health and well being of an organism. Vital energy is the by-product of nourishing input, strong digestion, and the elimination of toxic residues. Retaining substances that are meant for disposal creates disease. Effectively dispensing of waste products supports health by eliminating toxins and freeing up life energy consumed in the walling off of toxicity.

To eliminate accumulated toxicity, we first need to recognize that it is present. This is true on all levels of life—environmental, physical, and emotional. How do you know if there are toxins in your life? If you are not experiencing abundant vital energy on a consistent basis, you have unprocessed residues that need to be digested. Having recognized the toxicity, the next step is to neutralize it. If there is an environmental toxin, stop the production and distribution of it. If it is something over which you can exercise some personal control, stop exposing yourself to it. Then take steps to ensure that you are allowing only nourishing elements into your system.

We've explored the physical toxicity that can sap our vitality, but for most people the depleting toxins are not physical. Toxic emotions and toxic relationships are responsible for most of the energy depletion that inhibits our expression of vitality. Identifying and releasing toxic feelings are essential to restoring the integration between body, mind, and soul that allows for vital energy to flourish. This area is of such importance that I have devoted a substantial part of chapter 4, "Release Depleting Emotions, Cultivate Love," to identifying and releasing the mental toxicity that inhibits our experience of vitality.

Since we have been lightening our load of toxins in this chapter, let's take the next step—replenishing the body through nourishment.

Vital Energy Key #3

Feed Your Body,
Nourish Your Soul

Leave your potions in the chemist's crucible
if you can heal your patient with food. —HIPPOCRATES

Once a year on the Jewish High Holy Day Yom Kippur, I go twenty-four hours without eating. During this day of fasting, I have learned a lot about food. One observation to which anyone who has ever been on a diet will attest is that no matter what time of the day or night it is, we are bombarded with messages to eat something...now! Billboards, restaurant signs, magazines, and radio and television commercials are incessantly shouting at me to put something in my mouth. I may not be thinking about food, but show me a picture of a deep-dish pizza or describe a Ben and Jerry's sundae, and like one of Pavlov's dogs, my salivary glands begin to secrete and my stomach starts to grumble.

Remove me from these external cues, and I am able to commune with my inner hunger signals. When I make the commitment to go an entire day without eating, I start checking in with my appetite long before it actually begins calling my name. Am I hungry yet? I become aware of an emptiness in my gut hours before I feel genuine hunger pangs. As time passes, I enter a stage when I could eat if the opportunity presented itself, but the sensations of hunger drift in and out of my awareness like a conversation across the airplane aisle. But at some point my desire for food reaches a demanding level and my body clamors for attention and action. *Feed me!*

If I decide to ignore this basic physiological prompting, I have the opportunity to witness what happens to my appetite. The enjoyable sensations of hunger at first escalate to uncomfortable sensations of digestive distress, but if I consciously ignore them, they steadily fade into the background of my awareness. By the time I break my fast after a day without food, I am surprised at how quiet my appetite and digestive functions are. Rather than experiencing the ravenous hunger that was consuming my attention the day before, I actually have to kindle my appetite with lighter, appetizing foods.

The whole process is reminiscent of a fire. The intensity of the flame initially rises, but if there is no fuel to consume, the fire fades to glowing cinders. If I wish to rekindle the flames, I need to add dry tinder, for throwing a heavy log onto the smoldering embers will either smother the fire or generate a lot of smoke. This analogy was not lost on the ancient Ayurvedic sages who thousands of years ago observed that a person's health was dependent upon his or her ability to digest the world. They introduced the concept of agni, which is generally translated as "digestive fire." The root of our English word "ignite," *agni* refers to the process by which we extract nourishment from our environment and transform it into the substance of our minds and bodies. According to Ayurveda, if our agni is strong, we can convert poison into nectar; if our agni is weak, however, we convert nectar into poison.

Kindle Your Digestive Fire

Your appetite is an important sign of healthy digestive power. When I ask patients the question "How is your appetite?" the most common response I get is "too good." People who struggle with their weight think of their appetite as an insatiable monster, which left unchecked will consume anything edible within sight. A strong appetite, however, is an indication that the initial phase of digestion is healthy. One of the first physiological functions to become altered under stress is our appetite. Many people lose their appetites when they are facing emotional or physical challenges. Others eat more, not so much because they are feeling hungry but because they are feeling empty and trying to fill their inner void with food. A strong, balanced appetite is key to vital energy, for it starts the process of ingesting nourishment from the environment.

Carol was tired. Even upon awakening first thing in the morning she was exhausted. She was initially excited about moving back to her hometown to care for her elderly mother but, after just a couple of months, found that her energy was faltering. Although usually someone who liked to eat, Carol was deriving little pleasure from food and had to literally force herself to eat once a day.

When she consulted me, it was clear that she was depleted and depressed. She was concerned that she had not been eating properly and was hoping that a nutritional supplement would give her the energy she was missing. Rather than focusing solely on her diet, we explored the ways that she might be able to improve her digestive power so she would be able to extract the optimal nourishment from her food. She learned to tune in to her bodily signals of hunger and satiety, began practicing eating awareness, and started using agni-enhancing herbs. As her digestive power improved, she rediscovered a healthy relationship between her food and her vitality.

The body is the dynamic end product of DNA, orchestrating food-derived molecules around it. We create a healthy body when we are able to ingest and absorb the essential nutritional building blocks of food, build healthy tissues from the extracted elements, and eliminate those components that are unessential. Our digestive forces govern the breakdown of food into its fundamental constituents, the formation of biochemicals, cells, and tissues, and the elimination of waste products. When agni is performing its job, we experience energy, enthusiasm, and strong immunity. When it is not doing its job of efficiently extracting energy and information from our environment, we experience fatigue and become susceptible to illness.

Listening to Your Appetite

What can you do to optimize your digestive power? The first thing is to get in touch with your appetite. Right now place your hand over your stomach and ask yourself the question "How hungry am I?" Think about your appetite as a fuel gauge with zero representing empty and ten denoting filled to capacity. Most Americans have never run completely on empty, which is how you would feel if you had not eaten for a whole day. Most Americans have been at ten, which is how you feel after your third helping at Thanksgiving dinner. Although most people do not fill their gas tank when it is half empty just because it happens to be the day when they usually buy gas, most people eat even when they are not hungry just because it is time to eat.

We have learned from an early age to pay attention to external rather than internal cues regarding hunger. As a child you most likely heard the expression "Finish everything on your plate; there are children starving in India." In India, children are told to clear their platters because there are hungry kids in China, and Shanghai offspring are warned about deprivation in Harlem. In my household, dessert or going out to play after dinner was the reward for consuming every morsel that was placed in front of me. Well-meaning parents around the world encourage their children to eat, whether they are hungry or not. Considering how early we condition our children to ignore their internal signals of hunger and satiety, it is not surprising that recent statistics suggest that over a third of Americans are overweight.

Just as a weak fire will sputter when you throw a hefty log onto it, you will not efficiently digest food eaten when you are not really hungry. A strong appetite is the stimulus to produce and release salivary enzymes, hydrochloric acid, and the many digestive catalysts produced by your pancreas and liver. Start listening to and honoring your body's inner wisdom by paying attention to your appetite. Do not eat unless you are really hungry—a level of two or three on the appetite gauge. Stop eating when you are at a level of seven. Then wait until your hunger is strong again before you put food into your body.

Appetite Gauge

0	1	2	3	4	5	6	7	8	9	10
Starving	Hunger pains	Very hungry	Hungry	Could eat	Neutral	Could stop	Full	Uncom-fortable	Over-filled	Stuffed

How to Eat

Good nutrition is part chemistry and part artistry. I have been watching my infant girl, Sara, constructing herself from the breast milk of her mother. For the first four months of her life, she was exclusively transforming the vital liquid she was deriving from my wife, Pam, into her skin, muscle, bone, blood, liver, kidney, and brain cells. What is this product of lactation known as breast milk? It is the distillation of Pam's blood, a filtrate of the essential elements of her body. The apparent simplicity of a growing infant belies the amazing miracle of metamorphosing food into life.

Eating is a sacred act, and our digestion benefits from this acknowledgment. Each day I see people who feel they are not deriving the optimal nourishment from their food. They often spend time reading articles on vitamins and supplements, looking for the magic nutritional bullet to provide them with the energy they are lacking. In their search for the elixir of vitality, many people have forgotten the basic truth that for eating to fulfill the needs of body, mind, and soul, it needs to be a celebration of life. Take time preparing your meals to optimize their nourishing value. Shop for fresh ingredients, explore delicious new recipes, and eat your meals in a pleasant, uplifting environment. Honor your body's messages throughout the meal, and stop eating when you are comfortably satisfied.

Although sumptuous food nourishes us emotionally as well as physically, the primary purpose of eating is to sustain our physical sheath. Attempting to satisfy an emotional need with food will be unsuccessful because it simply is not possible to fill an emotional void with food. Although a piece of strawberry cheesecake may temporarily calm your turbulent heart after learning your lover was cheating on you, the soothing balm will be short-lived, and you will have consumed food that your body did not want or need. Consequently, you will likely be unprepared to metabolize the superfluous matter—only adding to the burden placed upon your digestive forces. Try not to punish your body in an effort to ease your emotional wounds.

Lighting the Fire

Herbs and spices can help awaken the digestive fire. In most cultures around the world, a variety of flavors helps to ensure that the appetite is both aroused and satisfied. Although we have a proud tradition of richly spiced foods, the average modern American diet tends to be less experimental and relatively limited in the tastes explored. To maximize your digestive function, try adding more bitter and spicy foods to your palate. Scientific studies have shown that bitter flavors stimulate the stomach to empty and the salivary juices to flow. Pungent spicy flavors kindle the appetite and digestive fire. If you have been feeling that your digestive power is weak, try this simple herbal apéritif before your meals to wake up your digestive system:

Herbal Apéritif

1 teaspoon of lemon juice
1 teaspoon of gingerroot juice
    or ½ teaspoon of grated fresh ginger
1 teaspoon of water
¼ teaspoon of honey
1 pinch of black pepper

YOUR MIND BODY APPETITE

Complete the following questionnaire to help identify your predominant digestive pattern. Choose the numbered response that best corresponds with your experience and tendencies.

SECTION 1	not me at all	me to some extent	definitely me
1. My digestion is on the slow side.	1	3	5
2. I often feel heavy after a meal.	1	3	5
3. I gain weight easily.	1	3	5
4. I have a tendency to overeat.	1	3	5
5. My bowels are usually regular.	1	3	5
6. I like to take my time eating a meal.	1	3	5
7. I sometimes eat out of boredom.	1	3	5
8. I have tried to diet at least once in the past year.	1	3	5
9. I feel drowsy after eating.	1	3	5
10. I believe I have a slow metabolism.	1	3	5

Section 1 Score _____46_____

SECTION 2	not me at all	me to some extent	definitely me
1. I have a strong appetite.	1	3	5
2. I can eat almost anything.	1	3	5
3. I get irritable if I am late for a meal.	1	3	5
4. My bowels are more likely to be loose than constipated.	1	3	5
5. I tend to get heartburn after eating spicy foods.	1	3	5
6. I occasionally have bleeding hemorrhoids.	1	3	5
7. I have a large capacity for food.	1	3	5
8. I use antacid medications at least several times per year.	1	3	5

Section 2 (cont.)	not me at all	me to some extent	definitely me
9. If I stay up late, I need to eat before going to bed.	1	3	5
10. I enjoy drinking milk.	1	3	5

Section 2 Score ____30____

Section 3	not me at all	me to some extent	definitely me
1. I have trouble digesting raw vegetables.	1	3	5
2. I sometimes forget to eat.	1	3	5
3. I often feel bloated after a meal.	1	3	5
4. I become anxious when I drink coffee.	1	3	5
5. I get constipated when I am stressed or when traveling.	1	3	5
6. I believe I pass more gas than most people.	1	3	5
7. I am sensitive to wheat or dairy products.	1	3	5
8. It is easier for me to lose weight than to gain weight.	1	3	5
9. I do not eat my meals at a set time.	1	3	5
10. I eat quickly.	1	3	5

Section 3 Score ____20____

MIND BODY APPETITE SCORES

Section 1 (Earth)   ____46____
Section 2 (Fire)   ____30____
Section 3 (Wind)   ____20____

Depending upon your mind body constitution, appetite and digestion may be more or less of an issue for you. Earth types tend to have sluggish appetites but eat out of habit and routine. Particularly if you have a tendency to gain weight easily, listen carefully to your body's hunger signals, and do not eat until you are really hungry. Fire types tend to have strong appetites, but under stress may experience hyperacidity with heartburn and indigestion. If you have a fiery constitution, do not allow the pressures of your day to delay your meals. Having your physical hunger satiated will reduce your likelihood of experiencing emotional overheating. Wind types tend to have irregular appetites, at times voracious and other times imperceptible. It is particularly important for people with a predominance of Wind in their constitution to stay in touch with their hunger signals and use herbs and foods to kindle the digestive fire. Honoring a healthy appetite is one of the most important components of a vital life.

Making Vital Energy Real

Awaken Your Fire

Listen to your body and honor its profound wisdom.
1. Pay attention to your appetite, eating only when you are hungry and stopping when you are comfortably full.
2. Eat your meals in a settled, comfortable environment, allowing yourself the time and space to focus on your food.
3. Take the time to shop for and prepare nutritious and delicious meals.
4. If your appetite or digestion has been weak, try the herbal apéritif before your meals.

Add Flavor to Your Life

My baby daughter is at the stage where she puts everything in her mouth. I am certain that she is recapitulating an evolutionary stage of humanity during which we orally sampled everything in our environment. How did we learn which foods were nourishing and which were potentially toxic? Although occasionally Mother Nature disguises her secrets, she has provided us with clues that we unravel through our sense of taste. If the orange sphere that you sample is sweet and juicy, it is a fairly good sign that it is okay to consume it in ample quantities. If, on the other hand, the leaf you bite into is so bitter it makes you grimace, it is pretty good evidence that it contains substances that are best avoided or consumed only in tiny amounts. Add the messages carried by the ten thousand or so smells distinguishable by the human olfactory system, and we have a lot of information by which to predict the nourishing or toxic value of a potential morsel.

The Ayurvedic seers of yore determined that foods could be categorized according to one or more of six primary tastes—sweet, sour, salty, pungent, bitter, or astringent. At first this scheme seems almost too simple, and yet Ayurveda, the timeless science of life, offers insights that are as applicable today as they were thousands of years ago. If all six tastes are available, you will feel satisfied and will have eaten a nutritionally balanced meal. You have probably had the experience of feeling full but not completely satisfied after eating a portion of food. This is usually due to a failure to include all six tastes in your meal. Paying attention to this simple principle can make the difference between a gratifying or unsatisfying diet. Let's look more closely at this scheme of six.

The Six Vital Tastes

Sweet

Most of what we consume on a daily basis falls into the sweet taste category, which includes all carbohydrates, proteins, and fats. Bread, pasta, milk, rice, nuts, potatoes, fish, fowl, and meat are classified as primarily sweet in taste. Fruits such as cherries, melons, and papayas also fall into the sweet taste category. If you look in your grocery basket at the checkout counter, the bulk of your shopping will include foods that are classified as sweet. The sweet category provides our major source of energy and encompasses much more than refined sugars, which should be consumed only in small quantities. Foods carrying the sweet taste provide the building blocks for the structural tissues of our body.

Sour

The sour taste is derived from organic acids. Citric acid, ascorbic acid, acetic acid, lactic acid, and oxalic acid are common sources of the sour flavor. Apples, citrus fruits, grapes, and berries are the richest source of the sour taste. Fermented foods such as vinegar, alcohol, aged cheeses, yogurt, pickles, and salad dressings are other everyday sources of sour. The sourness of oranges, grapefruits, strawberries, and tomatoes is due in large part to their vitamin C content, so by ensuring that these sour foods are present in your diet, you will be certain to have adequate amounts of this essential nutrient. Sour also stimulates the appetite and promotes digestion. A little bit of sour enhances the palatability of every meal.

Salty

Living systems are dependent upon salts, which are essential for regulating the electrical energy necessary for movement. Too much or too little salt can cause health concerns. In addition to adding flavor, the salty taste stimulates digestion and is mildly laxative and sedative. Most salt in our Western diet is in the form of table salt, but the salty taste is also found in many sauces, fish, seaweed-derived products, and soy sauce. A little bit of the saline taste enhances other flavors.

Pungent

The pungent taste is carried by aromatic essential oils found in peppers, onions, garlic, horseradish, ginger, and many other spices. We commonly refer to foods with pungent flavors as "hot," reflecting the heating effect these spicy foods have on our physiology. Pungent flavors increase appetite, stimulate digestion, mobilize secretions, and cause sweating. Many pungent medicinal herbs are useful for digestion and detoxification. American diets tend to be low in the pungent category, but a little bit of spicy fire is good for you.

Bitter

Although nobody actually likes the bitter taste, it can clear the palate and make other flavors taste better. It has a detoxifying effect on the body and helps to kindle the digestive fire. The bitter taste is primarily due to glycoside and alkaloid chemicals found in many plants, herbs, and spices. Green leafy vegetables are the most common source of the bitter taste, with certain greens, such as kale or endive, particularly acrid. Broccoli, eggplant, and asparagus are other good sources of the bitter taste. Most of the detoxifying and anti-inflammatory herbs such as aloe vera, gentian, goldenseal, and dandelion are substantially bitter in taste. Some bitterness is necessary to balance the other flavors.

Astringent

The astringent flavor is really more a sensation than a taste. The tannins that carry astringency cause a puckering of mucous membranes, creating a drying and compacting effect. Foods that are rich in the astringent taste include lentils, beans, fresh spinach, tea, honey, unripe bananas, and pomegranates. Increasing your intake of astringent foods provides expanded sources of fiber, complex carbohydrates, and healing plant chemicals.

Vital Meals

How do we use this information to create meals that will be sumptuous and nutritious and provide us with abundant vital energy? Paying attention to the six tastes fully satisfies these criteria. Consider these seven vegetarian meals. They are low-fat, high-fiber, rich in antioxidant vitamins, and fully balanced with the six tastes of Ayurveda.

American

Veggie burger on a whole wheat bun with tomato slices (sweet, sour, salty)
Mustard, relish, onions, pickles, ketchup (sour, pungent, sweet)

Endive, arugula, radishes, and cucumber salad with oil and vinegar dressing (bitter, pungent, sour)

Vegetarian chili (astringent, sour, pungent)

Chinese

Stir-fried pea pods, tofu, and water chestnuts with soy sauce (sweet, bitter, salty, sour)

Rice with raisins and turmeric (sweet, bitter, astringent)

Hot and sour soup (pungent, sour)

Green tea (astringent)

French

Spinach and ricotta cheese crepes with tarragon lemon sauce (bitter, astringent, sweet, sour)

Wild rice with mushrooms and onions (sweet, pungent, salty)

Butter lettuce with mandarin orange dressing (bitter, sour, sweet)

Fresh blueberries (sweet, sour, astringent)

Indian

Spinach and cottage cheese (sweet, astringent, bitter, salty)

Basmati rice with saffron (sweet, bitter)

Garbanzo beans with onions (sweet, pungent, astringent)

Yogurt with cucumbers and coriander (sour, sweet, pungent)

Italian

Spinach linguine (sweet)

Tomato sauce with zucchini, onions, mushrooms, and textured vegetable protein (sour, pungent, salty)

Spinach salad (bitter, astringent, sour)

Fava bean soup (astringent)

Strawberries with a dollop of whipped cream (sweet, sour)

Mexican

Black bean soup (astringent, sweet)

Fresh tomato salsa with chips (sour, pungent, sweet, salty)
Vegetarian fajitas with zucchini, peppers, onions, and tomatoes
    (bitter, pungent, sour)
Spicy rice with tomatoes and onions (sweet, pungent, sour)

Middle Eastern

Falafels, hummus, and pita bread (sweet, astringent)
Tomatoes, cucumbers, and yogurt (sour)
Greek salad with feta cheese, olives, red onions, and peppercinnis
    (bitter, salty, pungent)
Baklava with honey (sweet, astringent)

Making Vital Energy Real

Be Aware of the Six Tastes

It is not difficult to eat in a healthy manner, but it does require
some preparation and planning. Focus on ensuring that a variety
of foods and flavors are available at every meal. Notice how satisfied you feel when all six tastes—sweet, sour, salty, pungent, bitter, and astringent—are present. If you find yourself still hungry
after eating a full meal, check to see whether you have consumed
representatives from all taste groups.

Seek Nature's Nourishment

Plants have faced many of the same evolutionary challenges as
animals over the past several hundred or so million years. They
have had to adapt to changing temperatures, rainfall, atmospheric
conditions, predators, bacteria, fungi, and viruses. In their effort
to survive, our botanical cousins have developed thousands of
complex biochemicals, the vast majority of which we are only beginning to identify and characterize. These fascinating plant

chemicals, known as phytochemicals (*phyto* = plant), provide us with a wealth of potential healing substances that, hopefully, we will recognize before we decimate our environment and forever lose the flora that create them.

The most important news in nutrition over the past ten years is that there is more to food than calories, protein, fiber, vitamins, and minerals. Bioactive compounds found in fruits, vegetables, beans, and whole grains lower the risks of cancer and heart disease and strengthen our immunity. You may have been resisting the injunction to eat your broccoli since childhood, but we now know that a class of phytochemicals called isothiocyanates, abundant in broccoli, cabbage, and brussels sprouts, is very effective in detoxifying environmental carcinogens. Phenolic compounds, naturally present in tea, citrus fruits, grapes, and tomatoes, are antioxidants, strengthen blood vessels, and inhibit many carcinogens. Almost every fruit or vegetable you can consider is a natural health-promoting pharmacy in its own right.

Garlic, onions, leeks, and chives contain a chemical, allyl cysteine, which has a number of health-promoting benefits. Studies have suggested that people who consume these robust foods on a regular basis have lower cholesterol levels and lower blood pressure. Components of onions and garlic keep the blood-clotting cells, platelets, from becoming too sticky and enhance components of the immune system. Another chemical found in spicy foods, capsaicin, has a number of health benefits. This ingredient of hot chili peppers, black pepper, and cayenne has potent antioxidant properties, protects cells from cancer-causing substances, and can even act as a pain reliever when applied topically to the skin. Cooking with pungent foods not only adds to the flavor of your meal but may also enhance your health.

Other beneficial plant chemicals found in fruits and vegetables include bioflavonoids and lycopenes. Bioflavonoids, found in citrus fruits, berries, carrots, and broccoli, are mild antioxidants and seem to have a specific ability to block the effect of cancer-causing hormones. Lycopenes are present in tomatoes and red grapefruit and have a particular protective effect on the male prostate gland. In cultures where men consume large quantities of tomatoes in their diet, there is a markedly lower incidence of prostate cancer. Whether tomatoes are eaten off the vine, drunk as juice, or made into pasta sauce, they seem to confer a beneficial effect.

For many years it has been debated as to whether regular wine drinking is beneficial or harmful to health. Recent studies suggest that it may be something in the grapes rather than the alcohol that offers health benefits. A chemical called resveratrol is present primarily in the skins of grapes and has been shown to enhance the liver's detoxifying ability, block the effect of cancer-causing substances, and serve as an effective antioxidant. If you are striving to enhance your vitality, I recommend that you consume your daily dose of resveratrol in the form of a bunch of delicious red or green grapes each day rather than rationalizing your daily split of merlot.

Phytochemical	Common Source	Effects
Allyl cysteine	Garlic, onions, leeks, chives	Lowers blood pressure, reduces cholesterol, enhances immunity
Capsaicin	Chili peppers, cayenne, black pepper	Antioxidant, protects against carcinogens, topical pain reliever
Flavonoids	Citrus, tomatoes, berries, carrots, broccoli	Mild antioxidants, block cancer-promoting hormones
Lycopenes	Tomatoes, red grapefruit	Block damaging effects of radiation, inhibit prostate cancer
Resveratrol	Grapes (primarily the skin)	Antioxidant, enhances liver detoxification, inhibits carcinogens

Phytoestrogens

A family of plant chemicals receiving a lot of positive attention these days is the phytoestrogens. Consuming foods rich in these natural substances seems to confer many health benefits, including reduced risks of breast and prostate cancer, heart disease, and osteoporosis. Phytoestrogens help lower blood cholesterol levels and reduce the uncomfortable symptoms of menopause. There are three main classes of phytoestrogens, and eating foods from all three is beneficial. Soybean-derived products have been studied most intensively to date, as we have discovered that countries where the intake of soy-based foods is much higher have a substantially lower incidence of breast and prostate cancer. Tofu, soy milk, textured vegetable protein, tempeh, and steamed soybeans are staples of many Asian countries but constitute a minimal portion of the average American diet. Other sources of health-enhancing phytoestrogens are grains and sprouts. Lignans, found in flaxseed, barley, and wheat, are potent antioxidants that help prevent the development of cancer cells. Coumestans, present in sprouted grains and beans, may help maintain healthy bones and be useful in the treatment of allergies. There is mounting evidence that adding phytoestrogen-rich foods to your diet will improve your health and well being, and I strongly encourage you to do so.

Phytoestrogens

Isoflavones	*Lignans*	*Coumestans*
Soy beans, chickpeas	Flaxseeds, whole cereals, legumes, cow's milk	Alfalfa sprouts, clover sprouts, licorice

Focus on Balance

Although the information on phytochemicals is fascinating, it may also create consternation that now you have to worry about the natural chemicals in your food as well as the fat, protein, vitamin, and mineral content. Fortunately, if you focus on a balanced diet that includes the six flavors, you will ensure that all the classes of healing chemicals are represented. The average American diet does not lack the sweet and salty tastes, but you can improve the quality of sweet foods by increasing your intake of fiber-rich

whole grains that promote digestive health. To get the most benefit from sour foods, favor tomatoes, berries, grapes, and citrus
fruits that are rich in antioxidant vitamins and detoxifying phytochemicals. The pungent taste, considered essential in kitchens
around the world from Latin America to India, is relatively neglected in the United States, but now that you know the health
benefits of onions, garlic, and chili peppers, spicy foods should become a regular part of your diet. Foods with the bitter taste provide low-calorie daily doses of many different phytochemicals and
are sorely needed in this society where obesity in the face of mal-
nutrition is so prevalent. Finally, accessing the astringent taste
through beans, grapes, and tea assures your intake of phytoestrogens, fiber, and phenolic compounds, all of which help reduce
your susceptibility to illness and enliven your vital energy.

Making Vital Energy Real

Vital Nutrition

Ensure that your meals are prepared with fresh organic ingredients, including all six tastes in each meal. Focus on the various
photochemical classes and see how many can be represented in
your diet. The American Cancer Society recommends eating a
minimum of five fruit and vegetable servings per day and esti-
mates that less than one in ten Americans meets this goals. Other
nutritionists believe that at least nine servings per day of fruits
and vegetables are required to get the optimal amounts of phytochemicals.

Track your intake today and see if you can consume at least
two healthy servings of each of the six tastes.

1. Recommended sweet tastes: whole grains, pastas, fresh fruits,
low-fat milk, low-fat cottage cheese
My intake of sweet tastes today:

_____

_____

2. Recommended sour tastes: citrus fruits, berries, tomatoes, grapes
My intake of sour tastes today:

_____

_____

3. Recommended salty tastes: sea salt, soy sauce, tamari, salted fish (used sparingly)
My intake of salty tastes today:

_____

_____

4. Recommended pungent tastes: hot peppers, onions, garlic, leeks
My intake of pungent tastes today:

_____

_____

5. Recommended bitter tastes: leafy greens, broccoli, cabbage, green pepper
My intake of bitter tastes today:

_____

_____

6. Recommended astringent tastes: soybean products, lentils, split peas, spinach, cranberries, tea
My intake of astringent tastes today:

_____

_____

Personalize Your Diet

Mark was chewing his way through several rolls of antacid tablets on a daily basis. Despite the fact that his business was finally turning around after a year of real challenge and his strained relationship with his wife was improving, his heartburn was continuing to act up after every meal. His family doctor prescribed a stomach acid blocker, but it had to be discontinued due to problems with his liver. He had been unable to identify any specific dietary trigger to his gastric distress, so he continued eating any food he craved.

After learning about the different mind body constitutional types, he clearly identified his predominant element as Fire. After following a Fire-pacifying diet for a month, his indigestion resolved, along with other mental and physical symptoms of overheating.

As we explored in chapter 1, everything in the world can be understood in terms of the three primary natural forces of Earth, Fire, and Wind. As the most tangible expression of the energy we ingest from the environment, food can be understood in terms of how it influences the matter, metabolism, and motion forces within our bodies. Food carries the energy of the three principles and can augment or diminish those forces in our bodies. Becoming conscious of the effects of food on our minds and bodies allows us to choose more consciously to eat in a manner that is balancing to our nature.

The Flavors of Earth, Fire, and Wind

I'm sure you've noticed the influence of food on your physical and emotional state. After eating spicy dishes at an Indian restaurant, your heartburn may act up or your bowels may become a little loose over the next twenty-four hours. After a rich Thanksgiving meal you may find yourself drifting off for a snooze between the main course and dessert. The constituents of our food become the essence of our bodies, and the biochemical juices that are released impact our state of awareness and emotions.

Ayurveda has taken it a few steps further, classifying each food according to its proportion of the six flavors and its influence on the three mind body principles. For each principle—Earth, Fire, and Wind—there are three tastes that increase the energy and three that pacify it. The Earth element is increased by foods that are sweet, sour, and salty, and is lightened by foods with the pungent, bitter, and astringent tastes. The Fire element is heated up by pungent, sour, and salty flavors, and cooled by sweet, bitter, and astringent tastes. The Wind element is agitated by pungent, bitter, and astringent flavors, and settled by sweet, sour, and salty tastes.

	Earth	Fire	Wind
Tastes that augment the principle	Sweet Sour Salty	Pungent Sour Salty	Bitter Pungent Astringent
Examples of foods	Whole milk, ice cream, oils, avocados	Chilies, lemons, ginger, vinegar, mustard	Salads, cabbage, beans
Tastes that pacify the principle	Pungent Bitter Astringent	Sweet Bitter Astringent	Sweet Sour Salty
Examples of foods	Spinach, broccoli, ginger, lentils	Milk, rice, cucumbers, melons, asparagus	Rice, pasta, bananas, honey, milk, nuts

You need not be compulsive in order to benefit from this information. If your body has accumulated excessive Earth as expressed by weight gain, congestion, and sluggishness, favor more spicy, bitter, and astringent foods that are high in nutrients and low in calories. Salads, greens, legumes, and pungent spices generate lightness and increase the digestive fire. If you are regularly feeling overheated as manifested by heartburn, inflammation, sweating, and irritation, reduce your intake of spicy, sour, and salty foods. If you are feeling ungrounded and having trouble maintaining your weight, favor that convey the sweet, sour, and salty tastes.

The better you understand the inherent energies in your mind body constitution and how foods influence your energy, the easier it is to choose a diet that is balancing, nourishing, and enhancing of your vital energy. If you grasp the basic qualities of the three forces of matter, metabolism, and motion, it is easy to remember the types of food that increase or decrease their predominance, and you will not need to memorize lists of foods to consume or avoid. The Earth element is heavy, cold, and viscous, so foods that are light, warm, and dry are balancing. Lighter vegetables, including broccoli, cabbage, and celery, and lighter grains such as barley can help to balance the heaviness of Earth. Foods that are hot in both temperature and spiciness are beneficial for Earth types. Almost all spices except for salt are useful in balancing Earth, with cayenne, ginger, pepper, and garlic of particular value. Reducing the intake of heavy, thick foods such as cheese, ice cream, and most oils will contribute to a balanced Earth constitution.

The Fire element is hot, acidic, and intense, so foods that are cooling and bland will help turn down the heat. Cilantro, most greens, cauliflower, and fresh peas have a cooling effect on the system. Milk and mild cheeses along with rice and wheat can help neutralize the sour acidity of the Fire element. Certain spices are cooler than most, such as coriander, fennel, mint, and turmeric, and they can be used freely by people with a predominance of Fire in their constitution.

The Wind element is light, dry, and cold, so heavier, richer, warm foods have the necessary energetic characteristics to pacify the turbulent tendencies of people who are predominantly windy. Warm, thick soups, casseroles, and pasta dishes are generally balancing for Wind types. Milk, taken heated and spiced with cardamom or nutmeg, can help to calm the blustery Wind element. Hotter spices, including ginger, cinnamon, and garlic, can help warm and improve the circulation of Wind people. Those with a predominance of Wind in their nature tend to have more delicate digestions and need to be prudent in their use of spices. Cumin and coriander may be better tolerated than cayenne or horseradish. A summary of foods to favor and reduce to balance your mind body constitution is provided here. Remember that a vitality-enhancing nutritional program is not about straining. It is about acknowledging and honoring your uniqueness in order to access your inner reservoir of vital energy. These recommendations are designed to be balancing, not restricting. Consume foods from all the taste groups while favoring those that are more appropriate for your mind body nature. Use these suggestions as a guide while honoring your body's intelligence. Good nutrition depends upon the experience of eating as a celebration.

	To pacify Earth	*To pacify Fire*	*To pacify Wind*
Basic Guidelines	Favor: light, dry, warm foods; pungent, bitter, and astringent tastes	Favor: cool foods and liquids; sweet, bitter, and astringent tastes	Favor: warm, oily, heavy foods; sweet, sour, and salty tastes
Dairy	Favor: low- or nonfat milk Reduce: all other dairy	Favor: milk, butter in moderation Reduce: yogurt, cheese, sour cream	Favor: all dairy
Fruits	Favor: apples, pears Reduce: bananas, avocados, coconuts, melons	Favor: grapes, melons, cherries, apples, ripe oranges Reduce: grapefruits, sour berries	Favor: avocados, bananas, cherries, mangos Reduce: apples, pears, cranberries
Vegetables	Favor: all vegetables except sweet potatoes, avocados	Reduce: tomatoes, peppers, onions	Reduce: sprouts, cabbage
Sweeteners	Favor: honey Reduce: all other sweeteners	Favor: all sweeteners except molasses	Favor: all sweeteners
Oils	Favor: almond, sunflower in small quantities Reduce: all others	Favor: olive, sunflower, coconut Reduce: sesame, almond, corn	Favor: all oils
Spices	Favor: all spices Reduce: salt	Favor: coriander, cumin, fennel Reduce: hot spices like ginger, pepper, mustard seed	Favor: cardamom, cumin, ginger, cinnamon, salt, cloves, mustard seed, black pepper

Making Vital Energy Real

Eating for Your Mind Body Nature

Without straining, pay attention to those foods and flavors that are better suited to your mind body constitution. Ensuring that you have all six tastes available at each meal, notice how you feel when you consume flavors that are pacifying or augmenting to a particular mind body principle. If your body has accumulated an excessive amount of the Earth element, try following an Earth-reducing dietary program and notice a sense of increasing lightness. If you have been overheated in body and mind, follow a Fire-pacifying program and notice a subtle cooling of your physiology. If you have been having difficulty maintaining your weight because of a weak appetite or high metabolism, follow a Wind-calming dietary program and see if you experience more groundedness.

Use Herbs and Vitamins Wisely

We are witnessing an amazing revival in the Western world. After almost a century of absolute faith in the medical-pharmaceutical-industrial complex as the source of all disease-relieving interventions, people are flocking in increasing numbers to more natural approaches. As a result, herbal and nutritional supplements are experiencing a meteoric rise in popularity.

The use of herbal medicines in Europe is well integrated into the medical mainstream, where over half of herbs are prescribed by medical doctors and more than one out of four nonprescription medicines are plant-based. As medical reports document the increasing use of herbal medicines throughout North America and the world, an expanding body of scientific research is confirming that many traditional herbal substances have demonstrable pharmacological and clinical benefits.

This does not imply that we can use plant-based medicines indiscriminately or abandon pharmaceutical agents. Herbs are generally subtler in their actions and do not usually exhibit the same potency as synthesized drugs. I like to think of herbs as providing a source of subtle nutrition that focuses more on restoring balance than on treating a specific disease process. However, some herbs do have potent biochemical effects and should be used selectively and respectfully. I often hear people suggest that because herbs are "natural" they are safe, but you only need to consider hemlock, poison ivy, and coca leaves to realize that natural substances can be both powerful and toxic. Every health-promoting approach has a role in the healing process, but it is critical that we understand the right use and anticipated efficacy of the intervention, whether it is a drug, surgical procedure, or nutritional herb.

For the past six months Rebecca was feeling drained. Due to an intense workload and a challenging personal relationship, she had been sleeping fitfully. Her digestion was off, and she was assaulted by migraine headaches several times per week. I was the latest visit on a pilgrimage that included doctors, therapists, and healers of many traditions and persuasions. Although she had benefited in some fashion from almost every healing encounter, the number of herbal and nutritional supplements she was taking dismayed me. I counted a total of sixteen bottles of medicinal substances that she was taking daily, most of which contained pills and tablets that were formulations of several to dozens of herbs. I calculated that she was ingesting eighty-five different plant-based medicines each day. She did not know what most of the prescriptions contained and, sadly, reported that she had not noticed any real benefit from them.

Rebecca's story, while extreme, is not unique and raises several important points. If you are going to try an herbal approach, keep it simple. Allow yourself to experience the effects of a single herb or formula for a reasonable period of time. I generally recommend trying a plant-based medicine for six to eight weeks. If there is not an identifiable or measurable benefit by then, stop the herb and consider another approach. If you are taking too many things at the same time and have a negative side effect, it will be virtually impossible to identify the offending agent. Conversely, if you are taking twenty different supplements and feel some benefit, you may be consuming nineteen more than you need. Another problem with multiherbal formulas is that it is unlikely that you will receive adequate doses of any herb contained within the recipe. In Rebecca's case, she was taking one herbal formula for her energy depletion that included twenty-eight different herbs in a 250-milligram tablet. It is highly unlikely that any of the herbs in such low doses would be efficacious, even if they were the appropriate medicine.

Plant-Based Medicines

I am not a believer in allopathic herbology. By this I mean I don't support the use of herbs merely to treat a person's symptoms without looking to the deeper cause. If you are feeling fatigued, you could drink a cup of coffee, which can be seen as a plant-based medicine to enhance energy. But as soon as the caffeine is metabolized, the fatigue returns and you'll probably feel more depleted than before you had the coffee. Particularly if you are taking herbal supplements in the hope that your fatigue or depression will respond, it is critical that you look to the underlying imbalances and address them on the levels of body, mind, and soul. With this preamble, let's look at the top seven plant-based medicines on my energy-enhancing list.

Ashwagandha (*Withania somnifera*)
Ashwagandha has been held in high esteem in the Ayurvedic herbal pharmacy as a premier rejuvenative for at least three thousand years. It is now organically grown in the United States, where it is sometimes known as winter cherry and is readily available through several major American herbal companies in 300- to 500-milligram tablets. The name *ashwagandha* is a Sanskrit word meaning "having the smell of a horse," describing the strong acrid odor of the freshly cut roots. This potent smell has been interpreted traditionally as an indicator of ashwagandha's powerful en-

ergy-providing properties. It has a long and glorious history in the Ayurvedic literature as a rejuvenative tonic for restoring strength, immunity, and vitality. It is nourishing and grounding, demonstrating particular value when the Wind element has been creating turbulence and exhaustion. Although it is energy enhancing, it has the effect of calming the mind and can be taken at bedtime to promote deep, restful sleep.

A number of studies have been performed on ashwagandha that have supported its traditional role as a stress-neutralizing tonic. In animal studies, ashwagandha has been shown to dampen the physiological changes caused by stress on the adrenal glands. In human beings, ashwagandha has shown an ability to speed reaction time and enhance mental processing in structured neuropsychological tests. Enhancement of immune function and potent antioxidant properties have also been demonstrated for this rejuvenative herb. For Wind-generated fatigue, ashwagandha is a valuable herbal friend.

Gotu kola or Brahmi (*Hydrocotyle asiatica, Bacopa monniera*)

The word *Brahmi* in Sanskrit means "that which enhances awareness (Brahman)." The Latin word for the brain, "cere*brum*," is derived from the same etymological roots. Two different plants in India have at one time or another been referred to as Brahmi, both of which have similar properties. *Hydrocotyle asiatica* has become popular in the West, where it is most commonly known as Indian pennywort or gotu kola. The fresh or dried leaves of this creeping plant are used to improve memory and vitality. It produces a calming state of mind and can enhance sound sleep if taken before bedtime. In Ayurveda it is considered one of the prime rejuvenatives for the mind and nervous system.

The other plant called Brahmi, *Bacopa monniera*, contains several unique chemical alkaloids. Recent studies have shown that some of these chemicals have specific effects on the neurochemistry of the brain that may explain Brahmi's traditional reputation as a brain tonic. Possessing potent antioxidants, Brahmi has immune-enhancing, anti-inflammatory, and wound-healing properties.

Gotu kola is now widely available in health food stores, where it is usually sold in one-third- to one-half-gram tablets. *Bacopa monniera* is not as well known yet in the West, but will soon be available from several American herbal companies. As a nutritional aid in sharpening the mind without generating agitation, Brahmi is a true botanical treasure.

Ginkgo *(Ginkgo biloba)*

Chinese physicians have prized the medicinal power of ginkgo for thousands of years. A standardized concentrated extract of the leaves of this ancient tree is currently one of the most widely used herbal remedies in Europe, where it is prescribed for problems ranging from ringing in the ears to dementia. Since a recent study in the *Journal of the American Medical Association* demonstrated its efficacy in the treatment of Alzheimer's disease, ginkgo has received more serious attention from American health care providers. This study was particularly impressive because it showed that in some patients with Alzheimer's disease, ginkgo not only stabilized, but actually improved, memory, an effect rarely seen in this common degenerative neurological illness. Ginkgo seems to have many health-promoting benefits, including reducing anxiety and enhancing immunity. It may even improve sexual function in people on antidepressant medications, acting like a natural and safe Viagra.

Ginkgo is a potent antioxidant that may protect against tissue damage in conditions ranging from frostbite to heart surgery. It has the remarkable ability to decrease anxiety while enhancing mental performance, unlike most anxiety drugs that commonly cause drowsiness and mental confusion. Ginkgo has been shown effective in relieving women's premenstrual symptoms of bloating and congestion and in protecting mountain climbers from the effects of high altitudes. The only reported side effect of this exceptional plant-based medicine is a very rare bleeding complication, suggesting that it should not be taken along with any type of blood-thinning medication. For people having difficulty focusing their minds, ginkgo may provide valuable support.

Ginseng *(Panax ginseng)*

Ginseng may be the most popular herb in the world, with its use in China dating back at least six thousand years. It has been considered a botanical paragon of healing traditions from Asia to America. Rather than being used to treat a specific disease, ginseng has traditionally been viewed as a source of subtle nourishment to improve energy and vitality. Studies over the past twenty-five years have suggested that ginseng has adaptogenic properties, meaning that it protects the body from the harmful effects of stress. In addition, it has pain-relieving effects and strengthens immune function. Ginseng is classically known as a rejuvenative tonic with a mythical reputation of enhancing sexual function. Scientific studies in males of species from mice to men have suggested there may be validity to these traditional claims. The use of ginseng has been shown to increase the number and motility of sperm in men. Chemical compounds derived from ginseng enhance the release of a natural substance known as nitric oxide (NO), which is important in penile erection. Stimulating the production of NO underlies the efficacy of the potency wonder drug, Viagra.

Ginseng enhances components of life in both men and women. Ginseng added to vitamins improves a person's sense of vitality and well being, but like most potent substances, ginseng should not be used indiscriminately. A 1979 report in the *Journal of the American Medical Association* warned about potential restlessness and sleeplessness in 20 percent of regular ginseng users. Although the study did not control for the use of caffeine, ginseng does have a mildly stimulating effect that some people may be more sensitive to than others. There is an appropriate indication for the use of every healing substance, and not every remedy is good for everyone. Ginseng is an excellent tonic herb for people with a predominant Earth nature in which it helps to energize the life force. It should be used cautiously if the Wind element is the liveliest principle in your mind body constitution, as the additional energy provided by ginseng may engender turbulence.

Guggul (*Commiphora mukul*)

A close relative of myrrh, guggul is derived from the resin of a small thorny bush. The sap of the bark contains many different chemicals, several of which are unique to this plant. It has been traditionally used in Ayurveda as a purifier and rejuvenative. When the body accumulates excessive toxicity (ama), guggul is recruited to cleanse the blood.

Many modern studies have given support to its traditional uses. In both animals and human beings, guggul has been shown to lower blood cholesterol and triglyceride levels. It has been found to have potent anti-inflammatory properties and can be helpful in a variety of rheumatic conditions. It has a somewhat heating quality, and should be used cautiously in people who have a predominance of Fire in their mind body nature, but it is an excellent vitality-enhancing herb for those with either Earth or Wind predominance. If you have been taking drugs, drinking too much alcohol, eating unhealthy fatty foods, or just feeling generally toxic, guggul is an excellent plant medicine to help clear the channels of circulation and allow your life energy to flow more freely. It is now widely available from a number of American herbal companies.

St. John's Wort (*Hypericum perforatum*)

The ancient Greeks recognized the medicinal value of these bright yellow flowers over two thousand years ago. Although St. John's wort has only recently arrived on the herbal scene in North America, it has been a very popular medicinal herb in Europe for the past fifteen years. Over seventy million daily doses of hypericum are consumed daily in Germany, where it outsells every pharmacological treatment for depression. Dozens of scientific studies have attested to its efficacy with exceedingly rare reports of side effects. People taking St. John's wort often report improved sleep, diminished anxiety, and reduced restlessness in addition to a lightening of mood. It has traditionally been used to enhance digestion, stimulate immunity, and treat infections, properties that are only beginning to be explored by Western medical scientists.

The name *St. John's wort* may have been given to acknowledge the flowering of the plant toward the end of June, around the time of John the Baptist's celebrated birthday. Another explanation for the name derives from the tiny black dots on the flower petals that turn deep red when rubbed between the fingers. It has been suggested that this color change symbolizes the blood that was spilled when St. John was decapitated by order of Herod's wife and daughter. Regardless of the origin of its name, scientific research is revealing that hypericum has a complex nature with several distinctive chemicals that act upon specific regions of the brain. In both animals and humans, St. John's wort has the ability to balance neurotransmitter levels at a potency equivalent to antidepressant drugs such as Elavil or Tofranil.

Side effects are uncommon and generally mild. Indigestion, allergic reactions, and tiredness are reported in a small percentage of people taking hypericum. Light-skinned animals that graze on St. John's wort have shown undue skin sensitivity to sunlight, but there has been only one reported case of a woman developing a sun-sensitive skin rash after taking hypericum for three years. Unlike some of the tricyclic antidepressants, hypericum does not appear to have any negative effects on the electrical conduction system of the heart. Overall, St. John's wort seems to be a genuine herbal gift that can be a subtle but powerful aid in reestablishing psychological and emotional balance.

Valerian (*Valeriana officinalis*)

This robust-smelling herb has been known since Roman times as an effective calming agent. Although in high concentrations it can be sedating, in usual doses it helps to quiet a turbulent mind without creating drowsiness. Two major classes of chemicals have been defined in valerian—the valepotriates and the sesquiterpenes, both of which have been shown to have calming effects through their interactions with the brain chemical gamma-aminobutyric acid (GABA). This is the same neurotransmitter that is important in the actions of standard anti-anxiety drugs such as Valium and Xanax.

In addition to its calming effects, valerian has traditionally been used as an antispasmodic agent to relieve digestive and menstrual cramping. Some studies have suggested that it may also help to reduce elevated blood pressure and migraine headaches. In an interesting older study from Germany, valerian was found to be calming for people with agitation and restlessness but actually stimulating for people who have problems with fatigue.

It is common for people who are not experiencing the vitality they desire to have difficulty sleeping at night due to emotional or physical distress. This sleeplessness perpetuates the daytime fatigue that increases the anguish. The calming effects of valerian can help to break the cycle and support the restoration of vitality.

For people whose nature is dominated by the Wind element, valerian can help quell the turbulence. As a temporary aid, valerian
is a valuable natural ally.

Be Smart about Herbs

What is the best way to use this information about herbal medicines? I hope you have not already gone to the health food store
and purchased seven bottles of herbs. My recommendation is to
consider your current situation and the healing profile of each
herb and decide if one of them really stands out for you as fulfilling a need you have. If you are having trouble focusing your mind,
you might consider a trial of ginkgo. If you are exhausted because
you are not sleeping well, consider a trial of valerian. If you are
aware of a low level of depression, consider trying St. John's wort.
Use the following chart to approach the use of these herbs ration-
ally. Discuss the use of any of these plant-based medicines with
your health care provider and keep it simple. Do not sacrifice
good nutrition for herbal allopathy.

Common name	Latin name	Therapeutic effects	Cautions	Usual dosage	Time to see effect
Ashwagandha (Winter cherry)	*Withania somnifera*	Adaptogen (stress protector)	Mildly heating	⅓ to ½ gram twice daily	1 to 2 months
Brahmi (Gotu kola)	*Hydrocotyle asiatica, Bacopa monniera*	Mental tonic	Rare skin rash	⅓ to ½ gram twice daily	1 to 2 months
Ginkgo	*Ginkgo biloba*	Memory enhancer	Avoid if on blood thinners	40 to 60 milligrams twice daily	2 to 6 months
Ginseng	*Panax ginseng*	Tonic	May cause restlessness	¼ to ½ gram twice daily	1 to 2 months
Guggul	*Commiphora mukul*	Detoxifier	Gastric irritation	½ to 1 gram twice daily	2 to 4 months

Common name	Latin name	Therapeutic effects	Cautions	Usual dosage	Time to see effect
St. John's wort	*Hypericum perforatum*	Mood elevator	Rare photo-sensitivity	300 milli-grams three times daily	4 to 8 weeks
Valerian	*Valeriana officinalis*	Mental calmer	Sedating in high doses	$\frac{1}{3}$ to $\frac{1}{2}$ gram at bedtime	1 to 2 weeks

The Essentials of Vitamins

At least several times a week patients will ask me if I believe in vitamins. My customary answer is that I acknowledge our fundamental requirement for these basic nutrients but doubt that Nature had in mind for us to consume our nutritional requirements through a handful of gelatin capsules. The usual response to this statement is that our food supply is being grown, processed, and cooked in such a nutritionally depleting manner that we now need supplemental nutrients just to break even. I don't know if this is true, but I do know that organically grown foods are increasingly available, and if prepared with love and attention, they can provide nourishment for body, mind, and soul.

On the other hand, there are times in life when our need for nutrition may exceed our capacity to nourish ourselves. If you are facing or recovering from a serious illness, have had a suppressed appetite due to physical or emotional distress, are under inordinate stress, are in training for a challenging athletic competition, have been consuming alcohol or recreational chemicals, or have simply not been eating well, taking nutritional supplements may be prudent. In terms of health promotion and disease prevention, every vitamin, mineral, and trace element is essential. Scurvy, pellagra, and beriberi are rare these days because we have recognized the need for vitamin C, niacin, and thiamine. Most vitamin intake requirements were originally defined by how much was necessary to prevent or eradicate a deficiency illness. We still have not

clearly defined the optimal intake of an essential nutrient to support the highest level of health. Given the wide spectrum between
absence of a disease and ideal health, it is worth reviewing some of
the latest information on the health-promoting value of some key
nutrients.

The Radical Vitamins -A, C, E, and Beta-carotene

In the last chapter we explored the role of free radicals, those noxious little chemicals that react with the nearest organic molecule.
Our body's ability to neutralize these is key to prevention of illness and promotion of health. The antioxidant vitamins are our
prime defenders against the ravages of oxidative stress and must
be abundant in our diet to fulfill their task. The question is
whether supplementing with antioxidant vitamins improves our
health. We know that people who follow diets rich in vitamins A,
C, E, and beta-carotene have lower incidences of cancer and heart
disease. It is less certain that taking antioxidant vitamin supplements provides the same benefits as a diet rich in fresh fruits, vegetables, and whole grains. Nevertheless, in view of the evidence
that supplemental antioxidants may confer some protection
against the free radical damage that plays a role in coronary artery
disease, cancer, Alzheimer's disease, Parkinson's disease, and a host
of other degenerative disorders, it is easier to be an advocate than
a critic of antioxidant vitamins.

The need for antioxidant vitamins may increase as we age. A
recent study in the *Journal of the American Medical Association*
found that vitamin E supplementation in a group of people over
the age of sixty-five led to significant improvements in important
components of immune function. Recent studies have also suggested that vitamins E and C may reduce the risk of mental decline as we age. Perhaps the most important information that is
emerging is the suggestion that antioxidant vitamins work best
when all are present together. This is the way they are packaged in
nature, and this is how I recommend you take them if you are going to use supplements. My suggestion is that you find a good
antioxidant formula that contains all of the important free-radical-
fighting nutrients. If you are consuming abundant beta-carotene,
you do not need to take extra vitamin A, for beta-carotene is auto-

matically converted into vitamin A. Take your antioxidant formula with your main meal of the day, but do not replace good food with good supplements. A recent USDA study brings home this point. Two-thirds of a cup of blueberries provides more antioxidant potential that the recommended daily doses of vitamins C and E. The message is clear: first eat your fruits and vegetables; then take your vitamins.

Antioxidant Nutrient	Common Food Sources	Recommended Daily Allowance (RDA)	Recommended Supplementation
Vitamin C	Citrus fruits, tomatoes, green peppers, green leafy vegetables	60 milligrams	$\frac{1}{2}$ to 1 gram
Vitamin E	Safflower oil, whole grains, green leafy vegetables, nuts	15 IU	200 to 300 IU
Beta-carotene	Carrots, squash, cantaloupe, peas, apricots, cherries	None established	15 milligrams (25,000 IU)
Vitamin A	Milk, yellow and dark green vegetables, orange fruits	5000 IU	Derived from beta-carotene. You do not need to supplement separately.

Vitamins and the Heart

In addition to the preventive value of vitamins C and E on the heart, there is some fascinating information on the role of folic acid and vitamin B_6 (pyridoxine) in protecting against coronary artery disease. Several studies have now shown that an elevated blood level of an amino acid called homocysteine is associated with an increased risk of atherosclerosis. Increasing your intake of folate and B_6 results in a lowering of homocysteine levels and may confer protection against heart disease. Foods rich in these essential nutrients are listed below. Supplementation with a multiple vitamin that contains all the Bs may offer additional protection.

Folate-Rich Foods	*B_6-Rich Foods*
Dark green leafy vegetables	Fish
Asparagus	Soybeans
Broccoli	Bananas
Beets	Cabbage
Orange juice	Potatoes
Wheat germ	Prunes
Whole grain cereals and breads	Whole grain cereals and breads

Making Vital Energy Real

Respect Your Nutritional Allies

1. Consider a plant-based medicine to boost your vitality while you are integrating other body, mind, and spirit approaches. Have realistic expectations from the herbal product, and discuss your plans with your health care provider.
2. If you feel nutritionally depleted, consider supplementing your diet with a balanced multivitamin and antioxidant complex. Give the herb or supplement enough time (usually one to six months) to assess whether you are feeling benefit from the substance.
3. Most important, keep it simple.

Other Nutrients

If you read any books or magazines about diet and nutrition, you are aware of the steady flow of nutritional substances that step into the limelight as the current solution to fatigue, aging, and illness. Blue-green algae, grape seed extract, pycnogenol, quercetin, coenzyme Q10, DHEA, carnitine—these are just a few of the many nutritional substances that are promoted to improve health. Although there is usually a rational basis to support the potential benefit for each of these supplements, the clinical evidence is usually sparse, and the assessment of possible side effects is generally lacking. For these reasons I am not a strong advocate of nutritional micromanagement. If you are interested in exploring the benefits of a specific nutritional product, try it for a specified period of time and determine whether it is giving you the benefits you anticipated. Do not sacrifice time and attention spent on choosing and preparing nutritious meals in search of the latest magical nutritional extract.

As Hippocrates said, "Let food be your medicine and medicine be your food." In this way you can access the infinite organizational and integrative power of nature, rather than having to calculate the complex nutrient formulas necessary for optimal health and vitality. Use the wisdom of your mind and body, and you will find the natural, balanced path to a nutritional program that awakens and refreshes your vital energy.

Vital Energy Key #4

Release Depleting Emotions, Cultivate Love

They love as though they will someday hate
and hate as though they will someday love. —ARISTOTLE

Mental turbulence depletes our vitality. When we are caught in the turmoil of an agitated mind or heart, access to our vital energy reservoir is obscured. If you scuba dive, you know that stormy weather on the surface impairs visibility at deeper levels. Try closing your eyes and listening to the sounds around you. What do you hear? If the television is not blaring, you may become aware of the background noises in your environment—a car driving past on the street outside, a dog baying down the block, the refrigerator humming in the kitchen. Continue listening and notice that even in the midst of outer quietness, your inner activity disturbs the silence. We call these inner sounds thoughts. As the German philosopher Martin Heidegger pointed out, "Thinking is a subtle form of hearing."

Our thoughts and emotions are the very substance of our inner lives, and they are capable of energizing or depleting us. Learning to transform our thoughts and emotions is key to creating more vitality. We must unburden our hearts of the pains and disappointments from the past so we can live more fully in the present moment. Every impediment removed from your heart opens a channel for love to flow.

New modes of thinking and feeling lead to limitless possibilities. If you continue thinking and reacting in your familiar and accustomed ways, you will continue to experience the same reality. If you are satisfied with the reality you are experiencing, there is no reason to change your life. If, however, you sense you are not enjoying the gift of life to the fullest extent possible, I want to convince you that you can do something about it.

Be Flexible

Your experience of life is one of many possible ways to perceive and interpret the world. We can think of reality as the conversations we are having with ourselves describing our experiences. This dialogue is generated as a result of our perceptions and interpretations. If we want to see changes in our lives, we need to change our perceptions and interpretations. Each of us has his or her own pattern of scanning and filtering energy and information from the environment, based both upon our inheritance and learning. There are physiological limits to our sensory receptors that place boundaries on our perceptions. Unlike my beagle, I cannot hear sounds above twenty thousand vibrations per second. Unlike a honeybee, I cannot perceive ultraviolet radiation. Even within our species, we have wide differences in our perceptual abilities. Some people are naturally more visual, whereas others are more auditory. If you were born color-blind, you will not respond to certain frequencies of visual light that might be attractive or repulsive to another person. If you have a high-frequency hearing loss, your experience of a concert or a conversation will be different from that of someone who does not have that limitation.

Describe Your Reality

My reality is different from yours, in part because I perceive my world differently from you, but more important because I *describe* my experiences differently. Recall a recent event in your life. Notice how, as you are remembering the occurrence, you are selectively describing some aspects of the situation while leaving out others. You may recall how so-and-so looked and what they said when such-and-such a situation occurred. Your description of the event will be different from another person's story because you each select a different aspect of a situation to focus on. When I meet new people, I may primarily pay attention to what they are saying and how they are saying it. You may pay more attention to how they look, what they are wearing, or how they carry themselves. Because there is an immeasurable amount of information available to us at every moment, we *have* to be selective about what we allow into our conscious awareness.

In our quest for recapturing vitality, it is important to recognize that your emotional reactions are often the essential component of your interpretation of a situation. What is your heart telling you? What do you *feel* about the occurrence? Your emotional response adds the flavor that identifies your specific viewpoint of every event. Your experience of reality is the combination of your emotional charge woven into your internal conversation.

I saw a couple in consultation recently who related one of their recent arguments to me. Married for almost thirty years, they admitted that this quarrel was similar to hundreds they had engaged in over the course of their lives together. For years she had been struggling with multiple sclerosis and was increasingly troubled by fatigue. He had recently taken early retirement and was spending most of his days at home. Their argument ostensibly centered on a dairy-free diet she had been following. He suggested that she was feeling tired because of her restrictive nutritional program, which he believed was protein-deficient. She responded that her exhaustion had worsened since he retired because she had to take care of his needs throughout the day. You can imagine the hornet's nest that was subsequently stirred up. Although they may not have completely agreed on the precise history of events, they entirely disputed the legitimacy of each other's emotional reactions.

I am repeatedly fascinated by how deeply committed we are to our realities. The man in this couple clung tightly to his point of view that he was only trying to help his wife, believing that she was surrendering her authority to experts who were not offering any real benefits. From the wife's perspective, the issue was entirely about manipulation. She refused to accept the possibility that her husband had any motivation other than trying to control her. As a detached observer, it was easy for me to see that there was some validity to each person's perspective and that there were many other possible ways of looking at the issue. Getting this couple to accept and act upon these possibilities after thirty years of patterned behavior would be challenging, requiring a genuine commitment to change on their part. Fortunately, they had such a commitment and, over time, learned healthier ways to express their needs. The fruits of their willingness to change were deeper love and respect for one another. In order to transform established patterns of behavior, we need to bring the light of conscious awareness into the murky waters from which our behavior arises.

Embrace Diversity

Why do we hold so tightly to our viewpoints? The simple answer is that our limited perspectives are safe and familiar, even if they are not particularly fulfilling or evolutionary. It is easier to be right than to explore the possibility that there may be different or better ways of interpreting a situation. Since you have read to this point, I'll make the assumption that you are at least open to the prospect that there may be other ways to perceive and interpret your world.

If you accept the premise that your reality is one of many ways to perceive and interpret the world, spending your energy attempting to change someone else's perspective through argument or intimidation is a waste of your vital energy. The door to change always opens from the inside. Squandering your life energy trying to break down another's point of view will inevitably create more resistance and stifle love. You may succeed in temporarily controlling the other's behavior, but the effort expended in trying to dominate the person will sooner or later exhaust you. Spending your energy defending your perspective from someone else's onslaughts is equally fruitless. Relationships in which you repeatedly are in power struggles inevitably deplete both participants. Delicate hearts are bruised, and defenses are mobilized. We must transform wasteful energy exchanges into loving, nurturing ones.

When our thinking binds us to some particular limited perspective, usually rich in judgment and poor in tolerance, we often attract other people into our lives who are resonating on the same level. The more tightly I am bound to my position, the more likely I am to draw in people who are equally attached to a polar conviction. This does not mean that we should stop having strong feelings about anything. We simply need to be conscious of our perspectives, choosing those that are most likely to bring happiness to ourselves and those affected by us. Becoming conscious means recognizing that we are metabolizing every experience in the present moment flavored by our past experiences.

If my heart was wounded in second grade by a red-headed girl with freckles, I may be carrying a pocket of unprocessed hurt that gets stirred up every time I encounter a woman with red hair. In the stirring of these feelings, I will search for and identify bits of information that reinforce my expectation that red-haired women cause me pain. We are continuously selecting what we pay attention to and how we interpret the experience. When we realize that we are choosing our perceptions and interpretations, we can loosen our rigid attachment to a limited, unproductive viewpoint and shift our focus away from people who drain us of our vitality.

Don't Waste Your Energy

Most of us have had the experience of going to a movie with a friend, expecting to enjoy the show and the company. During the film you may have become entranced with the characters and plot but noticed that your friend was yawning frequently throughout the picture. After the show you expressed how engaging you found the film, while your friend complained that it was trite and predictable. What is the reality? It was clearly different for each person.

We each wear a set of filters through which we screen our experiences. Based on our mind body nature, our filters provide a unique hue to our inner and outer worlds and determine how we handle our differences with others. When your view of the world conflicts with another person's reality, the way you manage those differences can either augment or deplete your vital energy.

If you have a predominance of Earth in your nature, you probably try to avoid confrontation, seeking to overlook differences. If this tendency is excessive, you may be reluctant to express your opinions or state your point of view for fear of engendering disagreement. Although on the surface this lack of resistance may seem virtuous, people who fear confrontation often hold in their feelings and are eventually depleted of vitality.

Fiery people, on the other hand, have a low threshold for expressing their judgment, at times demeaning others who have differing viewpoints. Although there is value in openly expressing one's feelings, the intimidating style of imbalanced Fire types may cause others to withdraw out of fear of being hurt or abused. People who cannot control their fire eventually scorch their own territory and burn up their vitality in the process.

Wind types are most likely to doubt their own reality, believing that people who appear self-assured have a more direct connection to the truth. Of course, the ultimate truth is that each person's reality is valid for that person. For those with a predominance of Wind in their nature, looking for guidance from within and learning to access their inner quiet voice are essential to tapping into the ocean of vital energy.

The secret to vitality is integration. Each and every approach to reality provides a piece of the puzzle. The Earth impulse to look beyond diversity, the Fire drive to discern, and the Wind tendency to change can all be valuable in deepening our connection to the source of energy and creativity that transcends the paths. The most important principle of a vital life is not to waste your life force. If you find yourself repeatedly expending energy defending your perspective or attempting to convince, cajole, or dominate another person, stop and recognize that you are squandering your energy. The great German novelist Thomas Mann told us, "We are most likely to get angry and excited in opposition to some idea when we ourselves are not quite certain of our own position and are inwardly tempted to take the other side." Although spirited debate can be exhilarating for some, ongoing conflict and arguing are depleting for everyone. Understand your nature, access your quiet inner voice of wisdom, and relinquish your need to attack or defend. It is only from this platform that genuine love can flow.

Making Vital Energy Real

Practice Flexibility

1. Notice each time you find yourself defending your point of view. Pay attention to how earnestly both you and the person with whom you are debating believe in the perspective being defended.
2. Develop an inner conversation of considering the other person's point of view. After a heated conversation, describe the discussion in your journal and acknowledge any valid points in the other person's viewpoint. Notice how this process loosens your attachment to a rigid perspective and lessens the intensity and frequency of energy-depleting arguments.
3. Become aware of how your mind body nature shapes your reaction patterns. Pay attention to your need for control or approval and practice relinquishing your attachment to the idea that your way is the only right way to see things.

Look into the Mirror of Relationships

How do we become more conscious of our choices and stop our inner monologue of judgment and defensiveness? By recognizing that all points of view are available within our own awareness. Try the following exercise to demonstrate this principle.

Identify something you feel strongly about. It can be an issue, a cause, a belief, an opinion, or a conviction. Now consider someone who opposes your point of view. It may be a public or personal figure. Having identified your antagonist, list the qualities that this person expresses that irritate you. See if you can come up with at least five or six traits you find really annoying. Now that you have identified what you don't appreciate about this oppositional person in your life, see if you can recognize some aspect of each annoying quality you listed in your own behavior. If you are truly honest with yourself, you will see that on some level, you are actually similar to the person who exasperates you.

Here's an example of how it might work. You are a financial consultant in an investment company and are ready to quit your job because you cannot stomach your supervisor, who is caustic, patronizing, demeaning, crude, and manipulative. He gets you so upset at times that you feel like smashing your computer screen and screaming. He is a petty tyrant, and despite your stated desire of getting as far away from him as possible, you end up taking him home with you every night in your mind. Look at each of his qualities that stir you up and ask yourself, "Do I ever express similar traits?" Your first reaction may be "Absolutely not!" but I would encourage you to go deeper and see if you can recall a time when you were caustic or manipulative.

The more you are able to embrace a highly charged quality in your own life, the less likely you are to be triggered by other people who are expressing that characteristic. It has been my personal and professional experience that the more strongly we deny a negative quality in ourselves, the more likely we are to express that trait in our relationships. If you have identified a characteristic in your antagonist that you just don't see in yourself, try asking a close friend who is willing to be honest with you. One of the best ways to determine whether you are denying an aspect of your nature that you don't wish to acknowledge is to ask, "Have you ever known me to be...?" As an example you might ask, "Have you ever known me to be demeaning? Do you ever feel I'm manipulative?" If you have created safety for your friend to be honest, you will usually learn that the trait you so strongly resist is within you, just below the surface.

The great psychiatrist Carl Jung was a courageous explorer of the hidden aspects of human personality, referred to as the shadow. He spent a good part of his life revealing the universal truth that we are multifaceted beings with many different aspects to our personality. We carry within our awareness heroes and villains, saints and sinners, loving, doting parents, and screaming, needy children. These internal characters are the basis of our creativity, richness, and mythology. Unrecognized, they are also the basis of emotional turbulence and suffering.

I urge you to become familiar with the diverse sides to your nature. Accept and embrace the different faces you wear. When you can love the various characters within your own being, you will spontaneously find yourself tolerating and appreciating a much wider spectrum of people around you. Recognizing the paradoxical components of your humanity does not make you weak—it makes you complete.

Reintegrate Your Shadow

Why do we reject parts of our being, relegating these abandoned characters to shadowland? Because we have learned that certain qualities are acceptable and others are not. I saw two people in my practice today who demonstrated how we lose our power when we deny essential aspects of our nature. A woman in her middle forties was raised in Russia but had spent the past ten years in the United States. She had recently separated from her husband of twenty years and her two teenage children because she did not feel she could grow in the marriage. When she first left her family she felt a wave of exhilaration as she stepped out on her own for the first time in her life, renting an apartment and starting a new job at a local library. She had visions of taking writing classes and traveling, but within a couple of months found herself nearly paralyzed with indecision. She had two voices battling in her mind. One was driving her to start over, make a clean break, and enjoy herself with carefree abandon. The other voice was longing for the security and safety of her family life. It was easy to imagine a little girl inside this middle-aged woman, pleading to have some fun, only to be told to be more responsible. She did not even consider the possibility of fulfilling her needs by creating opportunities for the different aspects of her being.

The second patient I saw today also demonstrated the sabotaging power of the unacknowledged shadow. This young man in his late twenties complained of fatigue and chronic back pain. Although he was an avid bodybuilder and well buffed, he projected very little personal power. He related that every time he started a project that had the potential for success, he lost interest and eventually undermined himself. Inquiring into his personal history, I learned that his father had left when he was ten years old. This young man had little memory of the circumstances leading to the breakup of his family but was quick to say that he did not harbor any ill feelings toward his father. He had never engaged in any conscious processing of his feelings about his abandonment. My interpretation of his story is that in his unconscious effort to wall off childhood pain and anger, he also blocked access to his source of vitality.

Meeting the Shadows of Earth, Fire, and Wind

Knowing the energies that predominate in your mind body nature can help you identify the hidden aspects of your being. Accessing the power of your shadow side can provide you with energy that had previously been unavailable.

Earth beings cherish stability and consistency in thought, word, and deed. The shadow side of Earth encompasses the opposite values of change and dynamism. The shadow side of Fire people includes those qualities that are not in control, unconcerned with power, and generally lighthearted and carefree. The shadow side of people dominated by Wind includes discipline, loyalty, and consistency. It is common to see Earth and Wind people developing relationships because each is attracted to the opposite qualities they express. In the beginning the Earth being is intrigued by the liveliness and variability of the Wind person, while the Wind person initially prizes the predictability and constancy of the Earth soul. A year later, the Earth person finds the Wind person to be flighty and unreliable, while the Earth being is seen by the Wind person as dull and boring. When the same qualities that attract you to someone subsequently annoy or repulse you, you are almost certainly dealing with your shadow. The more willing we are to explore the hidden aspects of our natures, the less we will need someone else to make us whole. When we try to fill the holes in our nature with someone outside ourselves, we are certain to be disappointed and project our frustration onto the other person.

If you are seeking a life rich with vitality, look into the mirror of relationships and openly and honestly explore what you see. Use the people who activate you both positively and negatively to look more deeply into your own soul and see what it is you are resisting and failing to acknowledge. By searching for the deeper meaning in every emotionally charged encounter, you will escape the prison of reactivity that depletes your vital energy. If you assume responsibility for your feelings and the people you attract into your life, you will achieve emotional freedom and the energy that it conveys. As both freedom and responsibility grow in your life, love moves into those places formerly inhabited by resentment and fear.

Making Vital Energy Real

Acknowledge the Positive and the Negative

Consider the most important positive and negative relationships in your life. Characterize the qualities in the people you love and the people you hate. Look at each quality that you find attractive and ask yourself, "How can I express this trait more in my life?" Look at each trait you find repulsive and ask yourself, "Is this a trait I deny in my personality?" Then see if you can identify a situation or circumstance in which you have demonstrated that quality. Simply acknowledging the positive and negative aspects of your nature helps you to be less reactive when encountering other people's idiosyncrasies. Notice how embracing the diverse aspects of yourself frees you to be emotionally available to the people in your life.

Person #1
Trait that I admire: How I can express this trait more in my life?
1. _____   _____
2. _____   _____
3. _____   _____

Person #2
Trait that I dislike: When or how have I expressed this trait in my life?
1. _____   _____
2. _____   _____
3. _____   _____

Create Emotional Balance

There are really only a few primary emotions. The most fundamental feeling is that of pain, and since pain hurts, we do everything in our power to avoid it. What causes pain? It is inevitably due to some infringement upon our boundaries of self. On a physical plane, we experience pain when the boundaries of our cells and tissues are breached by either internal or external assaults. Emotionally, we experience pain with loss (something that we feel belongs inside moves outside) or attack (something we feel belongs outside infringes upon our interior). When someone whose love or approval we seek does not provide it, we feel deprived and hurt. When someone criticizes, insults, or demeans us, we feel violated and hurt. Our heart closes down in a defensive effort to wall off the pain, and we deplete our vital energy in the process.

We react to emotional or physical wounding in two basic ways. Walter Cannon, a brilliant American physiologist in the first half of the twentieth century, described the fight-or-flight response. When an animal encounters a threatening situation, it responds by either being aggressive or retreating. If the animal believes it can win the battle, it will tend to fight. If it perceives its chances of losing are high, it will run away. To activate either of these life-preserving choices, we have evolved neurological and hormonal reactions. Our nervous system has a hard-wired stress response that causes our blood pressure to rise, our heart to beat faster and harder, our skin to sweat, and our adrenal glands to spurt out stress hormones. Our endocrine system releases a soup of hormones—cortisol, thyroid, glucagon, and more—that act like switches at a train station, diverting the energy of our body onto specific tracks. Although we rarely activate the full-blown fight-or-flight response in today's society, we do experience its emotional equivalents.

The emotional reactions of aggression or withdrawal are psychological equivalents of the fight-or-flight response. Most of us do not engage in a physical confrontation when our feelings are hurt; rather, we become intimidating and aggressive or withdrawn and remote. In simpler terms, we experience either anger or fear. Hurt, anger, and fear are the three primary colors of the emotional palette. Anger flares as a protective mechanism to discourage further incursions. Fear alerts us to the approaching danger and impels us to remove ourselves. These primary emotions are present in all of us, but we each have a propensity to react in a characteristic manner. One's individual repertoire of emotional reactivity has both inherited and acquired features. Some people by nature tend to respond aggressively to challenges, while others are more likely to withdraw. In either case, once emotional responses are activated, time must pass before the physiological changes subside.

Regaining Mind Body Balance

As we have been exploring, Ayurveda describes three different psychophysiological approaches to confronting life's challenges. If Earth dominates your nature, you will either take challenges in stride or tend to withdraw under the stress, depending upon how balanced or imbalanced you are. Like the earth, you move more slowly and are generally tolerant, but may have a tendency to be weighty and languid. Under chronic stress, you tend to go into hibernation, believing that you cannot mobilize the energy you need to change the situation.

If you have more Fire in your nature, you tend to respond to stress with irritability and anger. Like a fire-breathing dragon, you lash out when threatened, at times scalding the people in your life with your harshness. After releasing your frustration you feel better, but those around you, who have borne the brunt of your fury, need time to recover. A fiery nature allows you to accomplish your goals as you digest the world around you, but if you are out of balance, you may incinerate those people you love in the process.

If you are a person who tends to respond to stress in a Wind pattern, you will most likely become anxious and agitated when challenged. Your moods fluctuate as you consider and reconsider the various options in response to the threat facing you. Like the wind, movement and variability dominate your mind.

Take the following questionnaire to see where you fall within the emotional response framework of Earth, Fire, and Wind.

Section 1		*Characteristic of me . . .*			
	Not at all	Slightly	Somewhat	Moderately	Very
1. If hurt, I tend to keep it to myself.	1	2	3	4	5
2. It takes a lot for me to get upset.	1	2	3	4	5
3. I like my life to be routine.	1	2	3	4	5
4. I stay in bed when I am hurt.	1	2	3	4	5
5. I am good-natured and forgiving.	1	2	3	4	5

Total Section 1 Score _____

SECTION 2	*Characteristic of me . . .*				
	Not at all	*Slightly*	*Somewhat*	*Moderately*	*Very*
1. I have a tendency to control my relation-ships.	1	2	3	4	5
2. People perceive me as intense.	1	2	3	4	5
3. I get irritable when I encounter obstacles to achieving my goals.	1	2	3	4	5
4. I can be sarcastic or demeaning if someone disappoints or dis-respects me.	1	2	3	4	5
5. Patience is *not* one of my virtues.	1	2	3	4	5

Total Section 2 Score _____

SECTION 3					
1. I am prone to anxiety.	1	2	3	4	5
2. I am sensitive to the moods and opinions of others.	1	2	3	4	5
3. I tend to feel insecure in relationships.	1	2	3	4	5
4. I am a better talker than a listener.	1	2	3	4	5
5. Under stress, I tend to have insomnia.	1	2	3	4	5

Total Section 3 Score _____

MIND BODY BALANCE SCORES

Section 1 (Earth)   _____
Section 2 (Fire)   _____
Section 3 (Wind)   _____

Each of us has some aspects of all three psychological styles, but usually one or two predominate. Look at your highest score and see if you can identify your emotional response patterns. Pay attention to your expression of aggravated Earth, Wind, or Fire and learn to identify when you are deviating into a state of imbalance.

A Question of Balance

Our tendencies will be with us throughout our lifetimes. The secret to a vital life is how to channel our tendencies to cultivate maximum success, enjoyment, and love. When our daily choices and actions are consistent with our natural talents and propensities, we use our life energy efficiently. On the other hand, when we are constantly struggling against our natures, we waste energy and experience fatigue and exhaustion.

The concept of balance is an essential notion that pervades healing systems around the world. Western biologists and physiologists refer to the dynamic, self-regulating balance of living systems as homeostasis. In Ayurveda:

> A person whose basic emotional and physical tendencies are in balance,
> Whose digestive power is balanced,
> Whose bodily tissues, elimination functions and activities are in balance,
> And whose mind, senses and soul are filled with vitality...
> That person is said to be healthy.
>
> —Sushruta Samhita

When all aspects of our being—environment, senses, body, emotions, and spirit—are balanced and integrated, we are able to express our unique talents in ways that bring happiness, vitality, and success to ourselves and all those with whom we interact. For each trait and tendency that we possess, there is the potential for that quality to be expressed in either a life-supporting or a life-damaging way. From an Ayurvedic perspective, each psycho-physiological pattern—Earth, Fire, and Wind—can function in a balanced or imbalanced manner. One of the important goals of

Ayurveda is to identify areas of imbalance so we can make choices that reestablish balance.

The Earth element in balance leads to reliability, loyalty, and tolerance. When it is out of balance, dullness, lethargy, and stagnation arise. Loss of vitality in people who are Earth-element bound is due to excessive accumulation of toxic emotions and stagnant energy. Earth people hold onto things in their lives, including possessions, relationships, and emotions. Their path to vitality is through releasing unnecessary attachments to old wounds and obsolete emotional patterns.

A balanced Fire element radiates warmth, friendliness, intelligence, and competence. An imbalanced Fire principle generates excessive heat, leading to irritability and testiness. People whose Fire element is dominant lose their vitality by burning out. They set unrealistic goals and standards for themselves and others and become frustrated because they cannot achieve their objectives. In their emotional conflagration, they scorch the people closest to them and themselves. The recovery of Fire people is based upon choices that prevent their overheating in body and mind. They need to recognize when their fuse is being lit and remove themselves from the aggravating circumstance.

When the Wind element is operating in a healthy and balanced fashion, enthusiasm characterizes your life and you are engaging and energetic. You are flexible, open to new experiences, and comfortable with not being in control. When you are under stress, your Wind principle goes out of balance, and the qualities of movement and activity create turbulence. Your mind may become hyperactive, resulting in anxiety or insomnia. You may have difficulty completing tasks you have begun, lose your appetite, and be overly sensitive to your environment. Relating back to the primitive fight-or-flight response, Wind people are flighty. They cope with stress through activity and, left unchecked, become exhausted. To reestablish vitality, a Wind-oriented person must make choices that are grounding and stabilizing.

Operating from a state of balance enables us to express love to others. When we come from a place of imbalanced neediness, we often alienate the very people whose love we seek. Finding your emotional balance and opening your heart allow your vital energy to fulfill its intended purpose, intimately connecting you with other souls on the journey.

Making Vital Energy Real

Maintain Your Equilibrium

1. Witness the emotional reactions within and around you. Identify the primary ways in which you express your feelings, particularly when you are feeling pressured. When you see the energy becoming imbalanced, take a deep breath, bring your awareness back to your quiet inner state, and relinquish your attachment to the drama. You will more likely realize your intentions and desires if you remain established in your center.

2. Notice the emotional patterns of people in your environment. When you or someone around you shows evidence of restlessness, agitation, or nervousness, consider how the Wind element is aggravated. When you see irritability, sarcasm, or intimidation expressed, notice how the Fire element is flaring. When withholding, withdrawal, and denial are expressed, reflect upon the expression of imbalances in the Earth element. Become aware of these universal patterns ceaselessly expressing themselves in all aspects of your emotional life and focus on maintaining your balance amidst challenge and turbulence.

Observe the Laws of Your Emotions

How do we learn not to resort to maladaptive emotional responses? Despite what you may have learned in a weekend human potential seminar or in the latest popular psychology book, there are no simple answers to changing your core emotional patterns. For most of us, our reactions under stress are deeply embedded in the fabric of our personhood, with both inherited and learned components. We developed our patterns because they worked to some degree during times in our past. If, when you were four, your younger brother took your favorite toy away and by howling you got it back, you learned that expressing your anger could be effective in getting your needs met. If at age six, after being scolded by your mother, you hid in your closet, which caused her anguish until she found you and profusely apologized, you learned that withdrawing your love could be empowering. If you ran away whenever your parents started arguing, which forced them to stop fighting and focus on you, you learned the benefit of getting attention through flight. There are usually good reasons why we resort to our old standby responses.

The problem, of course, is that reactions that may have been useful when we were children are rarely as effective when used as adults. A tantrum at age two probably got your mom's attention, but this behavior at age thirty-two is unlikely to endear you to your family or coworkers. Taking your toys and running home after a disagreement with your neighborhood friend may have worked in kindergarten, but this pattern rarely nurtures an adult relationship. How do we transform our deepest emotional impulses to create vitality in our lives?

We don't usually think of our emotions as law-abiding, and yet as natural phenomena, our emotions are governed by universal principles, analogous to the laws of gravity or thermodynamics. The better we understand these basic principles, the more consciously we can choose to use our life energy for happiness and success rather than wasting it in ways that result in despair and disappointment. In the primitive soup of our emotions, there is a tremendous amount of raw energy that can empower or consume us. Emotions are deeply rooted in our evolutionary survival patterns, where they give us the strong impetus to seek food, defend our territory, escape danger, or form intimate bonds. Powerful physiological and chemical changes occur with emotional activation that can energize or deplete us, depending on how we use and are used by our feelings. Becoming conscious of the principles that underlie our daily lives can empower our inner worlds in the same way that uncovering the principles of gravitation and electromagnetism have transformed our outer world. Let's explore the five basic laws that apply to the realm of our emotions.

The Five Emotional Laws

1. I am ultimately responsible for my emotional life.
2. The setting of emotional boundaries with the appropriate balance of strength and flexibility is key to a vital life.
3. Emotional exchanges based on equality are energizing, while those that foster power imbalances are ultimately depleting to both parties.
4. The energy I expend avoiding my pain, denying my anger, and evading my fears depletes me of my vital life force.
5. Learning to embrace my uncomfortable and negative feelings enhances my capacity to experience the full depth and range of my vitalizing emotions.

Law #1   *I am ultimately responsible for my emotional life.*

This principle is often the most difficult one for many people to acknowledge. Emotions are so powerful it is easy to believe they have lives of their own and that we have little control over them. When someone says something rude or insulting, our reflexive upset seems fully justified as a direct result of the other person's behavior. "You hurt my feelings!" "You make me so angry!" "You make me feel worthless!" are the expressions we regularly use when others activate our emotions. We blame them for being insensitive, unappreciative, intimidating, and mean. We are generally not predisposed to recognize that the feelings generated are *our* feelings. Someone else may have activated the response by pushing the right emotional button, but the response is mine. On some level, our emotional turbulence is a choice, even though we rarely consider it this way.

There are, of course, degrees of responsibility in this choice-making process. If an alcoholic parent emotionally abuses a young child, we can hardly say that the child's deep emotional wounding is a conscious choice. However, as adults, most of us have established a pattern of predictable emotional reactions. If every time your boyfriend uses the word "bitch" you get very upset, you are making choices. If each time your mother uses the word "loser" you get upset, you are making choices. Placing yourself in situations that recurrently lead to wounded feelings is a choice. A more core choice is allowing the same hurtful words to consistently trigger your emotional reactions.

Think about a recent situation in which you became upset. Perhaps it was an argument with your boss, a phone conversation with your parent, or simply an encounter with a rude waitress. As you review the circumstance, notice the feelings that arise. If the incident is fairly fresh, you will probably experience many of the same emotions that arose when the original encounter occurred. Now recognize that these feelings are happening entirely within you. The discomfort arises as a result of how you are recalling and interpreting the original experience. You are generating the distress.

Now, shift your perspective. Consider the same situation from another point of view. In the case of our rude waitress, imagine a story that might place her behavior in context. She is a single mom raising her children, one of whom was sick this morning. This caused her to be late for work, resulting in her boss chewing her out right before you sat down for breakfast. When you complained about your toast being cold, she felt overwhelmed and responded curtly. You felt offended, but there were other possible responses, both then and now.

Hurt, anger, sadness, and fear are authentic emotions that will occur as long as we are alive. When we experience the unwelcome crossing of our personal boundaries, these basic emotions arise and are as natural to our emotional lives as our impulse to defend ourselves or withdraw from bodily assault. Responding openly and honestly at the time the situation is happening enables us to fully process the experience. Unfortunately, we are all laden with past impressions that color our perception and interpretation of every experience so that we are rarely responding solely to the situation at hand. Each new episode draws upon our history, so that we perceive the current situation through the filters of our past.

Your wife suggests you wear a different tie as you are getting ready to go out to dinner and you become irritated. You reject her advice, her feelings are hurt, and your evening is ruined. What happened? She believed she was offering helpful advice about your evening attire. In her family, her mother often helped her father choose his clothing. You interpreted her suggestion as disapproval, reflecting your early patterns with your mother. Your rejection of her counsel brought up her patterns of not being respected. A simple exchange stirs up lifelong issues.

Who is responsible for the upset? Each person is ultimately responsible for his or her own reactions. If the only way to avoid being swept up in emotional turbulence is for someone else to alter his or her behavior, you will forever be at the mercy of your environment. The energy wasted while you are jerked by the leash of your emotional reactions results in depletion and exhaustion. If you are truly committed to recovering your vitality, you must accept responsibility for your emotional life.

Law #2   The setting of emotional boundaries with the appropriate balance of strength and flexibility is key to a vital life.

We set boundaries to delineate our domain of control. Whether we are positioning guards at the borders of our country, a fence around our yard, or psychological defenses to protect our emotional well being, we set limits to define the territory over which we claim jurisdiction. When we feel our emotional sovereignty has been violated, we mobilize our psychological defense mechanisms and control dramas. We become upset, get angry, lash out, cry, deny, accuse, threaten, withdraw, throw a tantrum, mope, ruminate, become sarcastic, turn bitter, or resort to any number of other patterned responses that are within our particular psychological repertoire. Regardless of the specific reaction, the purpose is to reestablish a boundary that allows us to feel safe and in control of our own lives.

Your boss comes into your office and criticizes your job performance. Your defense mechanisms are activated, and you respond as you always have to intimidating authority figures. You may supplicate, cry, argue, or threaten to quit. You may feel hurt, angry, or anxious. You consider trying harder, garnering support from coworkers, thinking about quitting, or filing a lawsuit. Your feelings are legitimate, as are your reactions that reflect the best emotional response you are capable of mobilizing. The question is how you can expand your choices to maximize your sense of safety, empowerment, and fulfillment.

Boundaries are a necessary aspect of life, which when appropriately established provide value to everyone affected. When the boundary is breached, the energy expended should be sufficient to restore the lines without creating unnecessary repercussions. I once heard that overcompensation is a major cause of airplane crashes. I believe that overcompensation is also a major cause of emotional crashes. Setting your boundaries to provide the safety you require and responding proportionately to trespasses are the secrets to healthy emotional vitality.

How do we accomplish these goals? By paying close attention to the experiences that trigger our alarms. There is a classic Vedic story about the man who thought he had been bitten by a poisonous snake. He became so agitated that he began hyperventilating and was on the verge of passing out when an observer noticed that the "snake" was actually a piece of rope caught in a thorn bush. His interpretation of the provocation caused him much greater harm than the actual event.

This is frequently true for most of us. Time and again we get upset about a situation only to learn later that our interpretation was several degrees off. Time and again we find that our assumptions and projections have little to do with the reality of the situation. We make mountains out of molehills and create wars out of mild disagreements. And we waste a tremendous amount of our vital energy in the process.

Law #3   Emotional exchanges based on equality are energizing, while those that foster power imbalances are depleting to both parties.

We are a part of an infinite ocean of vitality. If we are not experiencing life energy flowing freely in our lives, it means that we are disconnected from our source, either giving it away or having it stolen. Although as children, we may have encountered people who were vitality thieves, as adults we are responsible for ensuring that all our interactions are primarily nourishing. Wilhelm

Reich suggested that love is the absence of anxiety. We can state it even more simply: love is the absence of fear. What are we afraid of? Having our boundaries trespassed, resulting in loss or invasion.

In the quest for recovering our vitality, we have to honestly assess each of our key relationships and ask the question—is this connection energizing or depleting? An energizing relationship is nourishing to both parties, because it is based upon mutual acceptance and naturalness. When we are engaged in a healthy loving relationship, we do not need to waste energy mobilizing our psychological defenses. A toxic relationship is based on control and manipulation, and it depletes both victim and villain. Although it may appear that the abuser is absconding with the power in the relationship, it is not really possible to take another's vitality—it is only possible to give it away.

Clara had been married to her husband for thirty-five years, the past ten of which had been hell. Her children had long ago given up encouraging her to leave the relationship, as she had an inventory of reasons why she could not. He controlled the money ...she couldn't manage the house alone...he knew where all the investments were. Despite the complete lack of love or respect in the marriage, she continued to tolerate his emotional abuse, believing that she had no other choice. When he died suddenly of a heart attack, all the responsibilities that she had so desperately feared became hers. To no one's surprise other than Clara's, she was able to competently shoulder the challenges and grew to enjoy the freedom that came with the responsibilities.

If you are waiting for someone else to change in order for you to feel better, be prepared to wait your entire life. If you want to regain your personal power from someone you perceive is stealing it, do not expect the thief to return it voluntarily. You must identify the needs that are being fulfilled by the relationship and seek alternative healthy ways to fulfill them. If you shift your perspective, the relationship will shift. If your partner is prepared to support a healthy transformation, your relationship will grow in intimacy, trust, and love. If the other person is not prepared to participate in the positive evolution of your relationship, you will more than likely grow apart. Pain is a warning signal from nature that something needs to change. If we fail to listen to the message that the pain is carrying, it will likely get more intense until we are forced to pay attention. I encourage you to listen carefully to the signals your inner being is sending and trust that your soul is guiding you to greater truth, wisdom, peace, and love.

Law #4   The energy I expend avoiding my pain, denying my anger, and evading my fears depletes me of my vital life force.

There are two primary sensations in life—pleasure and pain. It doesn't matter whether you are an amoeba or a nuclear physicist; the pleasure/pain principle is at the core of your being. When as a three-year-old child you trip and skin your knee, you automatically howl in discomfort, which mobilizes your mom or dad to come to your rescue and make it better. When a few years later your feelings get hurt because you are teased about being smaller, larger, plumper, skinnier, slower, more active, darker, or paler than your classmates, you learn not to show your pain, for it only makes you more vulnerable. If you suffered emotional, physical, or sexual abuse by a family member as you were growing up, you received pervasive messages about not expressing your pain or anger. We wall off our emotional pain like abscesses. Although the festering wounds may not be readily visible, they release a continuous stream of toxins preventing us from feeling vibrant and draining our vitality.

The classical psychoanalytic explanation of depression is that it is anger directed at yourself. You have been hurt but have been unable to adequately express your feelings because the consequences of showing your pain or anger seemed too great at the time. You were neglected or abused by a caregiver but feared that showing your distress would provoke them further. You were betrayed by a lover, but feared that setting an appropriate boundary would lead to abandonment. You tolerate your demeaning employer's rudeness because you cannot afford to lose the job. An appropriate outlet for your legitimate emotions is unavailable, so you turn them against yourself, resulting in depletion of your vital energy.

Inherent within any problem is its own solution. Honestly look at what you are feeling and ask the question "What am I *not* dealing with in my life?" Scan each of your important relationships and listen to the messages of comfort or discomfort your body is sending. If the message is one of distress, ask the next question: "What do I need to do to reduce or eliminate this distress?" Usually the answer is close to the surface and will burst into your conscious awareness simply by asking the question. For most non-nourishing relationships, you have three choices: change it, release it, or continue to suffer. Once you make your choices conscious, it is much more difficult to choose to suffer.

The next question is "What is preventing me from making the changes I know are necessary to recapture my vitality?" Listen to your responses, and be alert to the fact that this is usually where excuses and rationalizations arise. "I know I should change jobs, but..." "I know I should be more willing to express my needs in this relationship, but..." There are always plenty of reasons why it is easier to stay with the known than explore the unknown, but if the familiar is not bringing you the delight you deserve, you need to change your course or accept the consequences. Envision the event lines that flow from the choices you are considering, and remember that if you do not like the old script, you can write a new one.

Identify and release the burdens that are constricting your heart. You cannot change the past, but you can reinterpret it. Bear in mind that everyone is doing their best from their level of consciousness, although in retrospect we may wonder how a given choice was possible. Stop torturing yourself with recriminations and resentments. Do not compound the injury inflicted from without with inner blame. Seek to understand, relinquish your need to judge, and foster forgiveness. Carrying bitterness and hostility causes much greater harm to you than to the person at whom these feelings are directed.

Create a ritual of release. Write a letter, draw a picture, or take an old photo and empower it with the authority to discharge the toxic feelings you have been carrying. After expressing your emotions, tear up the object, burn it, or flush it down the toilet, symbolizing your release of the noxious energy that has been limiting your happiness and creativity. Know that you deserve to be happy and that by releasing your pain, anger, and fear, you are reclaiming your birthright to love and be loved.

Law #5   Learning to embrace my uncomfortable and negative feelings enhances my capacity to experience the full depth and range of my vitalizing emotions.

Life is the coexistence of opposite values. When the Creator brought forth light out of darkness, the template for our universe was formed. Activity and silence, male and female, inhalation and exhalation, matter and antimatter, heaven and hell—our inner and outer worlds reflect the inextricable weaving together of polarities. We cannot know heat without cold, courage without fear, joy without sorrow. Within the domain of our emotions, the height of our ecstasy rises from the depth of our sorrow. To live a life of vitality, passion, meaning, and love, we must be willing to embrace all facets of our natures without judgment.

The path to vitality is the path to wholeness, which implies that we must embrace all the diverse aspects of our being. We are conglomerations of contradictions and ambiguities. If you consider yourself on a spiritual path, it is natural to want to eliminate parts of your nature that you judge to be profane. Recognizing that you are selfish, insecure, demanding, petty, prejudiced, controlling, and hypocritical is difficult enough. Considering your lifelong struggle to deny and suppress those negative parts of you, actually embracing and loving these components may seem an impossible task. And yet our quest for wholeness requires that we acknowledge our multifaceted magnificence, seeing all our aspects as sacred. If our emotional repertoire only allows us to be nice, sweet, and agreeable, we severely restrict both the range and depth of our life experiences. It has been my personal and professional experience that when we consciously embrace our selfish tendencies, we are freer to express our generosity. When we acknowledge our fears and insecurities, we become more capable of accessing our courage and confidence. When we are willing to feel our sorrow, our capacity for joy is expanded. The more able we are to accept our uncomfortable aspects, the greater freedom we gain to embrace our sacredness and to see it and love it in all those around us. Walt Whitman said it beautifully:

I am the poet of the Body and I am the poet of the Soul,
The pleasures of heaven are with me and the pains of hell are with me,
The first I graft and increase upon myself, the latter I translate into a
    new tongue.

Making Vital Energy Real

Make Use of the Laws

1. Make the commitment to take responsibility for your emotional life, remembering that responsibility means exercising your ability to have a creative response to your emotional triggers.
2. Evaluate your important relationships and ask if there are appropriate boundaries in place to support both safety and intimacy. If the answer is no, see what can be done to set appropriate emotional boundaries.
3. Look at each of your relationships in terms of balance of power. See if there are opportunities to reduce control issues and open to new levels of safety, trust, and intimacy.
4. Honestly look at the unprocessed emotional wounds you are nursing and embrace the feelings. Journal and express yourself, seeking professional help if needed. Make the commitment to release toxic emotions that are limiting your ability to experience nourishing love and intimacy in your life.
5. Embrace the many facets of your personality, both positive and negative. Give yourself the opportunity to experience the freedom that comes from recognizing that life is the coexistence of opposite values.

Metabolize Your Feelings

It is not uncommon for me to hear someone say, "I know I shouldn't let it upset me so much, but I can't do anything about my feelings." There is no question that our emotions represent a powerful and primitive aspect of our mental worlds. When we feel challenged or threatened, our nervous systems and endocrine systems release a burst of chemicals that activate our minds and bodies, overriding our rational perceptions. Until the chemicals are metabolized, our feelings predominate over any logical thought process. Recognizing that there is a life span to every emotion, our goal is to encourage the expression of the feeling so that it does not create lasting distress. To accomplish this, we need to allow the emotion to take its course while exploring how the feelings were triggered in the first place.

Try this exercise. Take a few deep breaths and, with each exhalation, release any tension you are holding in your body. Now allow your attention to float backward in time until you are able to identify a recent circumstance that provoked an emotional response within you. It doesn't have to be a major upset, just something that stirred you up or caused you some distress. Relive the upsetting incident as clearly as possible, noting the circumstance, what started it, what was said, how it ended, and how you felt during and after the incident. Now, cover the following points:

1. *Describe what you were feeling when you were emotionally activated.* In order to consciously influence emotional reactions, we need to begin the process of witnessing the surge of emotional energy that occurs when we get upset. As soon as you can while the upset is occurring, describe what it is that you are feeling. Do you feel hurt, invalidated, unappreciated, angry, disappointed, invaded, neglected, taken advantage of, abandoned, betrayed? By identifying the emotions that arise, you will begin to recognize your patterns of response. You may recurrently feel betrayed by people in your life. Someone else may routinely feel taken advantage by others. Another person may repeatedly feel disrespected. As you become conscious of your emotional reactions, you will notice that you express a limited set of responses that say much more about you than the people who trigger your wounded feelings.

2. *Identify where you feel the emotion in your body.* An emotion is the simultaneous experience of strong thoughts along with strong bodily sensations. We call our emotions *feelings* because we *feel*

them in our body. The heartache of loss or the gut-wrenching sensations of betrayal are not mere metaphors; we actually experience these emotions physically. Paying attention to the bodily sensations that comprise our emotions is key to fully processing them. When a strong feeling arises, shift your attention into your body and notice where it is located. Most of us feel our pain in either our chest or solar plexus. If you are less directly in touch with your emotions, you may experience emotional hurt in your head, neck, or back. Once you have identified the area of your body that is generating the feelings, allow yourself to fully experience the sensations, without attempting to resist or filter.

For thousands of years, it has been suggested that physical symptoms can reflect core emotional or life issues. A man who cannot bear his responsibilities develops back pain. A single mom who feels she is carrying the weight of the world develops neck and shoulder pain. An executive who feels his company kicked him in the gut when they transferred him develops a peptic ulcer. A woman who feels unappreciated in her role as wife and mother is diagnosed with uterine cancer. A man whose wife leaves him brokenhearted has a heart attack. Whether or not there is a scientific explanation for connecting our metaphors and the physical problems we develop, there is value in bringing our attention to the area of the body that is expressing itself and listening to the message it is sending. The more in tune we are with our physical layer, the earlier we will detect imbalances. The sooner we identify any impediment in the effortless flow of vital energy between body, mind, and soul, the easier it is to reestablish the connection.

Practicing body awareness will often generate emotional release. You may naturally find yourself moaning or groaning. Tears may flow or you may feel the urge to bellow or roar. Remember, emotions are primitive and powerful, reflecting millions of years of evolutionary development. Suppressing emotions requires life energy that is then unavailable for creativity, enjoyment, and love. Embracing the sensations in our body allows us to regain access to our primordial energy. Releasing trapped energy may also result in the alleviation of the physical symptom, if the process has not progressed too far.

3. *Direct your emotional energy into beneficial rather than harmful expressions.* As discussed earlier, the limbic system, a very ancient part of the human brain, governs memory, emotional arousal, and physical activation. When the limbic system is activated, we tap into our deepest evolutionary survival patterns, which through stimulation of our nervous and hormonal systems have enabled us to continue as a species despite a very threatening environment. When our emotions are triggered, our brains access ancient neurological networks that provoke us to respond vigorously to the perceived threat.

   We need to acknowledge the powerful chemical and physiological changes that occur when we become emotionally charged. Since physically acting out through fighting or escaping is usually not the most adaptive way to deal with the energy, we need to consciously release the pressure that is generated when we feel upset. We need to do something physical that does not harm others or ourselves.

   Take a brisk walk, go for a jog, ride your bicycle, pound a pillow, take an aerobics class, play a game of racquetball, dance to an old rock 'n' roll song, or hit a bucket of golf balls. Consciously breathe out the stagnant energy while you are doing something physically vigorous and observe the changes taking place in your mind and body. To effect change in our emotional patterns, we need to align our awareness with that aspect of our nature that is able to witness the agitation, but not be overwhelmed by it. Expressing ourselves physically allows the turbulence to dissipate, accelerating the recovery of our emotional balance.

4. *Explore why this particular incident emotionally triggered you.* It's fascinating how the smallest perceived trespasses can sometimes provoke a vigorous emotional response. A faint irritation in one's tone of voice, a subtle skeptical facial expression, or a slightly condescending body posture can provoke a cascade of feelings. Words, tone of voice, and body language are the tools of communication that can transmit appreciation or rejection,

respect or threat. When a word, tone, or gesture triggers an emotional reaction, we can use the experience to learn about ourselves. An emotional response provides the entrance to a trail that leads to an inner tangle of memory and emotion. If we can unscramble the messages, we can free up energy and creativity trapped in our psychic entanglements.

The most effective and empowering method that I have found for bringing clarity into pockets of emotional murkiness is to write about the experience. Recapitulate the situation, express your feelings, and be open to hidden associations that may rise to the surface. See the circumstance that triggered your reaction as an opportunity to learn more about yourself. By transforming a hurtful experience into a valuable life lesson, you lighten the burden of your heart.

You come home from work and your wife comments that you haven't gone on a vacation for over a year. You become irritated and respond by saying you couldn't possibly take off work now because you are so busy at the store. She reacts to your tone of voice, saying that she has also been working hard and could use a break. You quickly reach your limit, say you need a break right now, and storm out of the house.

Now the process begins. You start walking briskly while you go over the conversation in your mind. At first you are filled with righteous indignation as you ruminate about how unappreciated you feel. "Unappreciated…unappreciated…unappreciated." As this word reverberates in your mind like a mantra, it dawns on you that whenever your feelings are hurt, this word dominates your awareness. With the first impulse of witnessing, you become aware of the sensations in your solar plexus. You feel tightness in your stomach as if you have been kicked in the gut, and you recognize that the exchange of words with your wife has been translated into visceral sensations. You consciously release the tension you are carrying in your abdomen and take some deep cleansing breaths. You realize you have been feeling a lot of pressure in your life lately and haven't exercised in over a month. You start jogging, and as your tension relaxes, you begin to notice there is a world outside your mind. Your vision becomes less narrowly focused, and you start appreciating the spring flowers blooming around you and notice children playing outside with their dogs.

By the time you arrive home, you are a different person from when you left. You ask your wife for a few minutes alone before you talk. You begin writing about your experience, and while journaling, you recognize that whenever you are feeling overloaded, any suggestion that you should ease up rather than push ahead harder generates instant irritation. As you consider this emotional reflex, you recall times when you pushed yourself so hard you thought you were going to burst. You remember messages from your father or mother about "quitters are losers" and their disappointment in you whenever you did not come out on top. As you become conscious of this underlying inner conversation, it dawns on you that with business as good as it's been lately, you can afford to hire part-time help and you really would love to take a week off with your family.

The secret to living a vital life is to *live* a vital life. Our internal dialogue determines our reality and is ultimately our responsibility. We all know people who seem to have it all—family, a challenging job, material abundance—but who are constantly lamenting about what is missing. We may also know other people, perhaps with physical disabilities, who despite severe challenges prize each day of their lives as a supreme gift. Their hearts are open and they allow life to flow through them without resentment. If we are prepared to live consciously, we can use the gift of our emotions to gain access to previously closed corridors of our heart and soul that offer us the immeasurable gifts of freedom and wisdom.

5. *Translate your emotional insights into greater love, safety, and intimacy in your life.*

The real proof of an evolutionary change is how much better we deal with a challenge that previously consumed our life energy. If in the past, you invariably felt upset whenever your boyfriend commented on your weight, you expended a tremendous amount of your vital energy in being offended. Consciously or unconsciously, you taught your partner "Press this button for an emotional pyrotechnic display." If, as a result of your inner processing, you now feel much clearer about the knots that bound you up in insecurity, the next time the button is pressed, there will be no fireworks. You no longer waste your vital energy, either in defending your territory or in the explosion of your emotional land mines. Observe what happens the next time the issue comes up. Do you allow yourself to fall into your previous rut of fear-based reactivity, or do you deal directly and nondefensively by openly sharing your feelings without need for approval or validation? Moving beyond your usual reactive mode opens the possibility for love rather than fear to be expressed. Fear depletes vital energy. Love replenishes it.

Making Vital Energy Real

Process and Release

1. Practice the emotional release process whenever you experience an emotional upset. Identify what you are feeling, bring your attention into your body, and experience the sensations of the emotion. Perform some ritual of release and look for the deeper meaning of your emotional response.
2. Have it your clear intention to expand your emotional freedom in all your relationships by taking responsibility for your feelings and using the mirror of relationships as a tool to gain deeper insight into your heart.

If dealing with emotions was easy, most relationships would be nourishing, and divorce, abuse, and emotional distress would be rare experiences. The truth is that emotions express raw, passionate power that can be creative or destructive. If we wish to channel the energy of emotions in creative ways that are likely to generate enthusiasm, happiness, and love, we need to practice processing our feelings. There is a skill in living intimately with other people that takes attention and intention to develop.

The payoffs for doing this work are freedom and vitality. Freedom grows as we assume responsibility for our emotional lives and stop blaming those around us for how we feel. We stop waiting for others to change in order to be happy. Vitality expands as we free up the energy we have sequestered in holding on to resentments and regrets. To use a technical metaphor, the more space we free up on our emotional hard drive that has been occupied by stagnant feelings, the more availability we have to run new and improved emotional programs. For your sake and the welfare of all those you love and who love you, release your depleting emotions and open your heart to the present moment, so abundant in wonder, delight, and vital energy.

Vital Energy Key #5

Move to Nature's Beat

The heavens rejoice in motion...
—JOHN DONNE

Movement is the essential feature of life. The evolutionary flow of energy distinguishes biological beings from the molecules used to assemble living bodies. Healing traditions across time and cultures have identified this energy stream as the vital force that governs the flow of evolution. In traditional Chinese medicine, this life force circulating through subtle pathways in the body is called *chi*. The stagnation that results when the vital force is obstructed in its natural circulation leads to imbalance, illness, and ultimately death. In Ayurveda the essence of the life force is called *prana*, which translates as "the primary impulse." Prana is sometimes referred to as the vital breath highlighting the inextricable interweaving of life and respiration.

At a subtler level, life is not merely movement but rather movement with rhythm. Rhythm implies action alternating with stillness. Day and night, inspiration and expiration, kinetic and potential energy, activity and rest—these are the steps of evolution that sustain vitality. Each day in my office I see people who can neither effectively rest nor act. They are caught in an energy-depleting spiral, unable to perform dynamic activity due to fatigue or chronic pain and unable to gain the deep rest they need to rejuvenate their bodies, minds, and souls. They are out of sync with the rhythms of nature and have lost their ability to tap into the wellspring of rejuvenation. As a by-product of our technological mastery we have fallen out of step with the ancient timeless pulse of the cosmos and pay the price in terms of distress and fatigue. Fortunately, we only have to listen for, and tune in to, the timeless cosmic beat and we can recapture our vitality. Let's explore how.

Dance to the Music

As human beings we have millions of years of evolutionary intelligence woven into our genes. Every cell in our body is governed by cycles of rest and activity that developed in synchrony with the rhythms of nature. Our stomach cells secrete acid at regular and predictable times during the day. Our pituitary gland releases pulses of hormones with consistent peaks and troughs. Our liver, kidney, and bone marrow cells all have dependable on and off times during the day, following an unseen conductor that maintains the rhythm of our bodies. Honoring the inherent rhythmicity of life has been a feature of cultures around the world, but since the dawn of the technological age, we have tried our best to disavow any need to align with nature's cycles.

I recently saw an emergency room nurse in consultation who illustrates the extent to which we have forgotten the importance of maintaining rhythm in our lives. She had been working a twelve-hour night shift for over ten years, usually going to bed after her children left for school in the morning. Four months ago she began a twice-weekly real estate class that was held from nine to noon at a community college, so that two days each week she actually skipped sleeping altogether. Her digestion was irregular, and (surprise!) she was fatigued most of the time. Although she knew her lifestyle was less than ideal, she was hoping that there would be a simple solution such as an "energy herb" that would forestall the need for her to make any substantial changes in her circumstance. Like it or not, we can't fool Mother Nature that easily.

The good news is that it is not difficult to harmonize with the rhythms of nature because they are hardwired into our DNA. Our bodies intrinsically know when it is time to eat, rest, and act in order to experience optimal vitality. We simply need to listen to and honor the messages being transmitted from inner space and stop reacting like Pavlovian dogs to the environmental stimuli that bombard us. Let's see what the ancient sages tell us about creating harmony in our minds and bodies.

Early to Bed, Early to Rise: Honoring Chronobiology

Edison invented the electric light bulb in 1879. For hundreds of thousands of years prior to this invention human beings ignited wood, wax, or various flammable oils to extend the productive hours of their day. But without constant attention these burning light sources faded; I doubt that our prehistoric ancestors spent too many nights partying into the wee hours. Cable television shows, twenty-four-hour convenience stores, and all-night bars were in short supply, so on most days our ancestral family was sleeping within a few hours after sunset. Without plantation shutters to block the light or radio alarm clocks to arouse them in the mornings, our progenitors relied upon the light of the local star to signal the dawn of a new day.

Over the past century, with the advent of technology, we have gained the freedom to eat, sleep, and be entertained at any hour of the day or night. If I choose to, I can watch a midnight movie until two in the morning, heat up a frozen dinner for a 3 A.M. snack, and sleep in until noon. That evening I can board a jumbo jet and arrive within a day and a half in any time zone or climate I choose.

It seems that for the first time in the history of life on planet earth, we can ignore nature. We can, but there is a price to pay for this ignorance—depression and loss of vitality.

Over the past twenty years we have learned a lot about the science of biological rhythms. The field of study known as chronobiology (*chrono* = time) has revealed that healthy cells, tissues, and organisms require periods of rest and activity in order to maintain health and vitality. We carry within us an internal clock that governs a host of rhythms including sleep and wakefulness, fatigue and mental alertness. When our inner biological clocks are not aligned with the pulses of nature, we experience irritability, difficulty concentrating, and depression. An organism or cell that has lost its rhythmicity is an organism or cell in distress. Cancer cells, for example, lose the ability to regulate their periods of resting and replicating. As a consequence they cause havoc in the cells around them.

One of the most common expressions of rhythm loss among people is the experience of jet lag. When we rapidly travel across several time zones, we encounter a desynchronization between our inner clock and the rhythms of the new environment. Our sleep is interrupted, we feel irritable, we have trouble focusing our attention, we seem disoriented, our appetite becomes altered, our digestion and elimination are disrupted, and we may feel depressed. After a few days, we entrain with the rhythms of our environment, and the distressing symptoms subside. Researchers have attempted to shorten the time it requires to adjust to a new time zone through the use of melatonin or bright lights, but there is debate as to how successful these interventions are. It seems that it simply takes time for our inner clocks to reset.

People who chronically feel fatigued commonly express many of the symptoms of jet lag. It is as if their biological clocks are perpetually out of harmony with the rhythms of nature. See how many of these symptoms you have been feeling:

_____ Poor-quality sleep
_____ Irritability
_____ Difficulty concentrating
_____ Disorientation

_____ Poor appetite
_____ Weak digestion
_____ Irregular elimination
_____ Depression

In my experience, many people troubled with the above complaints will show dramatic improvement in their overall quality of life by following a better daily routine. An ideal daily routine, known in Ayurveda as *Dinacharya*, is key to a healthy and vital life. Let's see what this ideal routine might look like.

Ideal Daily Routine

Morning

Awaken at sunrise

For those of you used to watching late-night movies until two in the morning, the thought of rising and shining at dawn may elicit audible groans. And yet, if you get into the habit of awakening with the sun, after just a few days you will notice a remarkable improvement in your quality of life. Do not use an alarm clock to rouse yourself, for starting the day with a stressful jolt does not set the right tone. Rather, keep the shades partially open so the light at daybreak can rouse you back to the waking state of consciousness. Earth types who need more rest will feel greater vitality if they get to bed earlier at night rather than sleeping late in the morning. Once you are awake, get out of bed and continue with your morning routine.

Morning hygiene

Most people are ready to empty their bladders immediately upon arising in the morning. According to Ayurveda, regularly evacuating both your bowels and bladder is important to maintaining good health. As a medical student I was taught that a daily bowel movement is not essential, but Ayurveda disagrees with this, suggesting that holding waste material longer than necessary is harmful to health. Many people I see lacking vitality have irregular digestive function, which gets worse under stress or when traveling. Normalizing elimination is an important component of recovering vital energy. To encourage this, try brushing your teeth first thing in the morning and then drinking a cup of hot water with a couple of slices of fresh gingerroot and lemon. This herbal tea has the effect of gently stimulating your bowels and promoting elimination.

Daily Massage

A daily oil self-massage followed by a bath or shower is a great way to get your energy circulating. The entire procedure need take only a few minutes, so there is really no excuse not to integrate one into your daily routine. Try the simple procedure described in chapter 2 each morning for a week and you will notice a profound change in your morning mood and energy level. A daily massage helps to soothe both the nervous and endocrine systems as the skin contains thousands of small nerve fibers and is a rich source of hormones and neurochemicals. Massage also enhances circulation and improves muscle tone.

According to Ayurveda, different massage oils are useful for different mind body types. Earth types benefit from lighter oils like sunflower, safflower, or mustard. Fire constitutions do best with cooling oils like coconut and olive. Wind types benefit most from warm, heavier oils like sesame and almond. Prior to performing a massage, the oil should be gently reheated above body temperature by placing a small quantity in a plastic cup or squeeze bottle and setting it into a bowl of very hot water. It is best to perform your massage in the bathroom, as no matter how careful you are, some oil may get spilled. To minimize this, use a plastic sheet to cover the floor or spread a large towel on the floor while doing the massage.

Doing a full-body massage sometimes takes too long for everyone's morning schedule, but massage is so beneficial that I would rather have you do a short massage than none at all. The most important parts of the body to cover are the head and feet. They can be worked while you sit on the edge of the tub for a minute in the morning. This mini-massage takes only about two tablespoons of oil.

Mini-Massage

Take one tablespoon of warm oil and rub it into your scalp, using small, circular motions. Massage the forehead from side to side with your palm. Gently massage your temples, using circular motions, then gently rub the outside of the ears. Then massage the back and front of your neck.

Taking the second tablespoon of oil, vigorously massage the soles of the feet with brisk back-and-forth motions of your palms. Work the oil around your toes with your fingertips. Sit quietly for a few seconds to relax and soak in the oil, then bathe normally.

Bathing

Keeping a thin, almost undetectable film of oil on the body is considered beneficial for toning the skin and for keeping the muscles warm during the day. Therefore, it's recommended that you wash yourself with warm water and mild soap. If you look good with glossy hair, leave a bit of oil on your scalp, but most people will need to use shampoo.

Stretching Exercises

Gentle stretching of your joints and muscles helps reduce stiffness, improve circulation, and enliven vital energy. I'll be offering a program to open the subtle channels of circulation later in this chapter. For now, know that a few minutes of gentle yoga is a great preparation for meditation.

Morning Meditation

Taking twenty to thirty minutes to calm and clear the mind through meditation is the most important component of a vitalizing daily routine. The technique you use should be effortless, whether it be watching your breath or silently chanting a mantra. If you have not been instructed in an effortless meditation technique, try the following one. It often helps to make a recording of the instructions in a slow, relaxing voice and then play it for yourself until the procedure is familiar to you.

Breathing Awareness Meditation

Sit comfortably with your eyes closed and your back supported. Take a few slow, deep abdominal breaths, releasing the tension in your body with each exhalation. After a few full inhalations, allow your breathing to return to normal and simply observe it with an innocent attitude. Witness the inhalation and exhalation of your breath without the intention to consciously alter it in any way. If you notice that your breathing changes, becoming faster or slower, shallower or deeper, do not resist the changes. Simply follow your breathing in this innocent, effortless manner.

When you notice your attention drifting away from your breath to another thought in your mind, a sensation in your body, or a sound in your environment, gently shift your attention back to your breathing. Relinquish your need to control this natural process. Now continue practicing this breathing meditation for about twenty minutes. When it is time to close the meditation, allow your awareness to float freely and continue with your eyes closed for a couple of minutes before beginning your morning activity.

Breakfast

Most of us have been taught that breakfast is the most important meal of the day. I am not sure that this is true. I do know that not everyone's digestive tract is ready to eat at seven in the morning. Eat breakfast when your appetite is strong, even if it doesn't happen until 10:00 A.M. After breakfast, take a short walk to aid your digestion.

Midday

Until the dawn of the Industrial Revolution, human beings ate their largest meal at midday. Studies have shown that our digestive juices are secreted in highest concentrations around noontime, which may explain why most preindustrial cultures favored a bigger midday meal and a smaller dinner. With the advent of assembly lines and typing pools, businesses could not afford to have employees take time off to eat their main meal during the workday. The consequences of this priority change are seen today in the many people who develop indigestion after a lunch that consists of wolfing down a sandwich while simultaneously taking a conference call and working through a spreadsheet.

One of the most important things you can do to improve your vitality and well being is to take the time to eat your lunch consciously. Even if it means spending only fifteen minutes, turn off your phone, warm up a meal, and focus on your food, using the conscious eating tools introduced in chapter 3. After lunch, try taking a five-minute walk to enhance digestion. A little activity after meals reduces the likelihood of post-eating drowsiness. If you consistently find yourself dozing off after a meal, try lying on your left side for a few minutes with your attention in your stomach. Even if you drift off for a couple of winks, you will awaken refreshed and energized.

Evening

Evening Meditation

Your second meditation of the day is best performed before your evening meal. Instead of a glass of wine or plopping down in front of the television, take twenty to thirty minutes of inner silence. The deep rest you gain will help to release the stress, settle the turbulence from the day, and rejuvenate you for your evening activities. If you fall asleep during your period of relaxation, spend a few minutes meditating before getting up to eat your dinner.

Dinner

Aim to eat your evening meal around six o'clock. Try to avoid eating a heavy dinner. This becomes increasingly important the closer you get to bedtime. Going to bed on a full stomach will substantially increase your chances of having a fitful rest. It will also enhance the likelihood of developing a powerful case of indigestion and may contribute to obesity. Wait at least two hours after a full meal before going to bed.

Evening Activities

To the extent that it is possible, keep your evening activities moderate. Particularly if you are having difficulties sleeping at night, avoid intense mental or physical effort in the evening. It's best to exercise in the morning after meditation or in the late afternoon before your evening meditation. If you perform intense activity too close to bedtime, your mind will continue to be dynamic when you want it to calm down. Rather than watching a violent action movie before bed, try viewing a nature show or light comedy. Go for a walk with your family, read a book, take a bath, write a letter, make love.

Bedtime

Deep, replenishing sleep is essential to regaining vitality. Insomnia is a widespread health problem around the world, and it tends to worsen as we age. Daytime fatigue as a consequence of poor sleep affects almost one in five adults and influences many aspects of a person's quality of life. Even our immune system is altered as a result of poor sleep.

I have found the following program very helpful in reestablishing a healthy sleep-wake cycle. If you are currently taking a medication to help you sleep, you can safely begin this natural sleep-enhancing regimen, but do not discontinue your medication without first discussing it with your health care provider.

How to Sleep Better

- Eat a relatively light dinner.
- Avoid exercise or intense mental activity after dinner.
- One hour before bedtime, spend ten minutes writing down the things that are creating anxiety for you and/or the things you have to do the next day.
- Perform a self-massage with warm oil a half-hour before bedtime.
- Take a warm bath with the lights low and soothing music playing.
- Add a calming essential aroma oil to the bath water or diffuse it in the air—lavender, vanilla, or sandalwood.
- Before brushing your teeth, drink a cup of soothing herbal tea—valerian, chamomile, mint—or drink a cup of hot milk to which ¼ teaspoon of nutmeg has been added.
- If you do not have a warm body to snuggle against, try using a heating pad or warm water bottle held to your solar plexus. Be careful that it is not so warm as to burn your skin.
- Once in bed, lie quietly with your eyes shut with your attention in your body, observing your breathing, counting each breath backwards from one hundred.

Most of the time, you will be snoozing before you count to ninety. If despite this process you continue to have trouble sleeping, try setting an alarm to awaken at 4:00 A.M. and do not allow yourself to take a nap during the day. Plan to be in bed by 10:00 P.M., and you will very likely be sleeping within minutes. If you awaken during the night, go to the bathroom, drink a half cup of hot milk or herbal tea, then return to bed and practice breathing awareness until you drift off. Performing vigorous physical exercise during the day will also facilitate restful sleep that night.

Your Mind Body Nature and Your Daily Routine

Depending upon the predominant elements in your constitution, it may be more or less difficult for you to align yourself with a vitality-enhancing daily routine. Earth types have the easiest time getting to bed early but have more difficulty getting up with the sun. They tend to be better at adhering to the resting, as opposed to the active, components of a routine. If you have a higher proportion of Earth in your nature, you will want to make certain that you perform some vigorous activity every day and are careful to listen to your body, eating only when you are really hungry and not just because it is mealtime.

Fire types are generally better at honoring their appetites and getting up early but have more difficulty turning off their day and getting to bed at a reasonable hour. Particularly if they are facing a project with a time deadline, Fire people will override all bodily signals of fatigue and keep pushing until the task is completed. If you have a predominance of Fire in your nature, you need to be careful not to burn your candle at both ends. Take time to rejuvenate before embarking on your next conquest.

Wind types have the most difficulty maintaining a healthy daily routine. Wind types easily find themselves in an imbalancing cycle as their nature inhibits them from following a regular routine, which only exacerbates the underlying turbulence. The stress of life results in increasing anxiety, insomnia, and digestive irregularities. Although it is difficult for Wind people to move to a steady beat, the extent to which they can maintain rhythm in their lives determines their mental and physical well being. If you have a predominance of Wind in your sails, recognize that bringing balance into your life will augment, not stifle, your vitality and enthusiasm.

Regardless of the major elements in your mind body nature, focus your attention on harmonizing your internal rhythms with those of your environment and you will experience greater harmony in all aspects of your life. We are spiritual, emotional, and physical beings. Honoring our biological rhythms enhances all the layers of our lives.

Making Vital Energy Real

Establish Your Rhythm

Commit to following an ideal daily routine for one week. Without being overly compulsive, try following a program that aligns your daily rhythms with those of nature. Even if you are only able to focus on just a few of these components, you will see an improvement in your vital energy.

1. Awaken at sunrise without an alarm clock.
2. Meditate in the morning.
3. Eat breakfast when you are hungry.
4. Make lunch the main meal of your day.
5. Take a short walk after eating.
6. Meditate in the late afternoon.
7. Eat a lighter dinner.
8. Perform light activity in the evening.
9. Be in bed with the lights off by 10:30 P.M.

Breathe into Vitality

The first thing we do when we arrive on this planet is inhale. The last thing we do when we leave is exhale. In between we respire about a half billion times, usually without any conscious attention.

The control center for respiration resides deep within our brainstem, where it is the most protected function in the body. Even when we lose consciousness, our respiratory center remains vigilant, faithfully monitoring our mental and physical state and governing the inflow and outflow of vital gases. There is an intimate relationship between our minds and our breath. The next time you find yourself emotionally upset, notice how your breathing reflects the turbulence you are experiencing. On the other end of the spectrum, many studies of people meditating have demonstrated that the breathing quiets down as mental activity calms.

The mind is a field of moving thoughts. When we choose to express our thoughts to the environment, we regulate our breath into words. Our breathing is influenced by our thoughts, and our thoughts can be influenced by breath. Learning to breathe consciously can be a valuable tool in helping to reestablish balance and vitality. As infants and young children we know how to breathe naturally and efficiently. As we get older, we learn to restrict the natural enthusiasm for life, which is reflected in our restricted breathing patterns. Rather than the easy abdominal breathing seen in infants, we learn to breathe primarily in our chests, where we hold stress and tension. Focusing on abdominal breathing takes advantage of the relaxation effect of using the diaphragm. When this muscular sheet at the base of the lungs contracts, it brings more blood and oxygen into the base of the lungs, improving respiratory efficiency. Upon relaxation of this muscle, the chest empties and we experience a sense of calm and comfort. Let's practice breathing in a more effortless, vitalizing way.

Abdominal Breathing

Find a comfortable sitting or lying position. Loosen your belt and remove any other restrictions that inhibit your belly from freely moving. Place one of your hands on your abdomen, just below your navel. Now take slow deep breaths into your belly so that your hand rises and falls with each inhalation and exhalation. With each exhalation contract your abdominal muscles slightly further to empty your lungs. Once you feel comfortable with this abdominal breathing process, remove your hand from your belly and continue taking slow deep breaths with your eyes closed.

As you are performing these slow deep abdominal breaths, try using a simple mantra to deepen your relaxation. On each inhalation, silently repeat the word "I." On the exhalation silently repeat the word "am." Continue with this pattern for several minutes, gently repeating "I...am...I...am...I...am..." with each respiratory cycle. If you want to try the traditional Sanskrit mantra, you can use the words "so" on each inhalation and "hum" on each exhalation.

You can use abdominal respiration whenever you notice you are restricted in your breathing. When under stress people often use only the top half of their lungs, barely moving their abdomen. When you find yourself restricting your breathing in this manner, consciously take a few slow deep abdominal breaths and release the tension you are carrying in your upper body.

Energizing Breathing

Just as we can use our breath to calm our minds and release tension from our bodies, we can use our breath to energize us. A breathing exercise from the yoga tradition, known as Bellows breath, is a powerful vitalizing procedure. Although it is generally a very safe technique, use this exercise cautiously if you have a known heart or lung disease. It is important that you stay tuned in to your body during this process. If you experience uncomfortable sensations, discontinue the breathing exercise for a few moments, then resume in a less intense manner.

Begin the procedure by sitting comfortably on the end of a chair. Relax your shoulders and begin practicing slow deep abdominal breathing. After a few deep breaths, fully exhale, then begin forceful complete exhalations followed by forceful deep inhalations through your nose at the rate of one full respiration per second. Perform ten deep breaths, then rest, feeling the sensations in your body. Wait fifteen to thirty seconds before repeating another round of ten complete breaths. Perform no more than three or four rounds at any one sitting. If you feel uncomfortably light-headed or experience tingling in your fingers or around your mouth, discontinue the deep breaths and simply observe your normal quiet breathing. Wait until the sensations completely subside; then try a cycle of only six to eight breaths. Your head, neck, and shoulders should remain relaxed, with the inhalations and exhalations coming from your diaphragm. The usual response after a breathing cycle is an experience of invigoration. This procedure is particularly useful if you have trouble getting going in the morning. Do not perform it after dinner, as you may have difficulty getting to sleep.

Empowering Breath

With your eyes closed, scan your body for areas of tension. Using slow deep breathing, release any pressure, resistance, or tension you are holding with each exhalation. Do this for about ten respirations. Now again scan your body and look for areas of weakness or vulnerability. You may feel this as a sense of emptiness or hollowness. People most often experience these sensations in the area around their heart or in their gut. If you are aware of an uncomfortable sense of visceral emptiness, the following breathing exercise can be very empowering.

Take a full deep breath, and on exhalation, audibly make the sound "Ahhhh" until you run out of air. As you express the sound, consciously direct the vibration into the area of emptiness in your body. If you feel delicate in your heart, see if you can vibrate your chest with the sound. If you feel a sense of emptiness in your solar plexus, allow the sound to resonate in your gut. Fill your body with the vibration, allowing the resonance to dislodge any toxicity you are holding and enliven the flow of energy. Repeat the sound several times at a sitting until you feel a sense of vitality. It can be performed for a few minutes prior to your meditation and can also be used while you are walking, gardening, or even waiting for an elevator (assuming you're alone). You may feel a little foolish the first time you try this exercise, but you will notice an empowering effect if you perform it regularly. You'll also notice how quickly your respiratory endurance improves both during the process and in all your activities.

I encourage you to play with these breathing techniques, experiencing for yourself their effects. Use them to help regain your balance and vitality. They are as low-tech as you can get and are always available.

Making Vital Energy Real

Vital Breathing

1. Practice each of the three breathing techniques and notice their influence on your mind and body. Use the abdominal breathing exercise when you need to calm your mind. Use the Bellows breath when you are feeling lethargic and need quick energy. Try the Ahhhh breath when you are feeling vulnerable and depleted.
2. Try substituting a breathing exercise for some other behavior that you would normally utilize. Try the abdominal breathing instead of taking an antianxiety or sleeping medicine. Try the Bellows breath instead of a strong cup of coffee. Try the Ahhhh breath instead of a couple of glasses of wine. Use your breath to enliven your body's natural healing pharmacy.

Stretch Your Limits

Wherever you are right now, don't move! Shift your attention to your body and notice how you are positioned. Is your body comfortable or uncomfortable? Can you imagine maintaining your current pose for the next fifteen minutes? One hour? Now, either sitting or standing, clasp your hands together and stretch them over your head for a few moments. Now how do you feel? Are you aware of a decrease in tension and an increase in energy? The simple act of stretching muscles, tendons, and joints can reset the balance point between tension and laxity and mobilize your life energy.

Loss of flexibility is an inherent feature of aging as our tissues become depleted of lubrication. From an Ayurvedic perspective, the longer we reside on this rotating planet, the more the Wind element increases, resulting in a gradual stiffening and dehydration of bodily tissues. To overcome this tendency, we need to stretch and mobilize our joints and muscles regularly. Every athlete knows that warming up before vigorous physical activity is critical to avoid injury. In a parallel way, stretching at the beginning of each day is key to maintaining long-term flexibility and avoiding the chronic pain that is so prevalent in our population.

Yoga—Conscious Stretching

The ancient system of yoga has gained acceptance in the West primarily as a series of physical postures. The word *yoga* comes from the same root as the word for *yoke*, as in yoking oxen, and ultimately the purpose of yoga is to unite body, mind, and soul. The physical poses that are the best-known component of yoga are most beneficial when performed with conscious body awareness. This means paying close attention to the sensations in your body while you are performing the posture rather than to the ultimate position you seek to reach. Yoga is not a competitive sport. Rather, it provides an opportunity to practice consciousness in motion. Maintain self-awareness while performing your yoga postures, and you will be increasingly able to maintain centered awareness in the midst of all your activities.

I have found it most useful to learn a basic set of yoga postures that you can practice on your own every day. If there is a yoga studio near you, I encourage you to take classes, but don't use the excuse of not being able to get to a class to avoid performing daily postures. Yoga does not need to be complicated to be effective. It simply needs to be performed consciously. Try the following seven postures while sitting in a chair, maintaining your awareness in your body and allowing your breath to flow smoothly throughout each position.

1. **Breath extension.** Sit comfortably with your eyes closed at 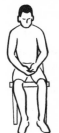 the edge of your chair without back support. Rest your hands in your lap with your shoulders relaxed. Now begin taking slow deep breaths, filling your chest with air. As you inhale, augment the extension of your spine by imagining that your head is rising up above your body. Feel the stretch in your rib cage and lower back. Hold your breath for a few moments at the peak of inhalation, fully lengthening your spine, then slowly exhale, allowing your body to slump gently. Repeat this process three times.

2. **Overhead stretch.** Raise your right arm slowly over your head, 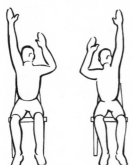 gently stretching at the shoulder. As you fully extend your arm, feel the stretch along your side. As you lower your right arm, raise your left arm over your head, stretching from the shoulder. Alternate one arm with the other, breathing easily with each extension. Repeat three to five times on each side.

3. **Forward fold.** With your hands over your head, slowly bend 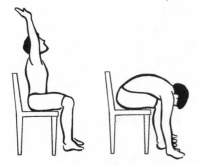 forward from the waist, gradually bringing your hands to the floor next to your feet. Let your head relax between your knees. Rest your abdomen on your thighs and breathe slowly and deeply, allowing your breath to massage your inner organs. After a few breaths, slowly come up one vertebra at a time, starting in your lower back and gradually working your way up to your neck.

4. **Side Twist.** Cross your right leg over your left thigh. Place

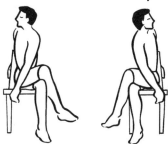

your left hand on your right thigh. Reach behind you with your right hand and grasp some part of the chair, using it to rotate your spine around to the right. Keep your head aligned with your spine and remember to breathe. Hold for a few respirations; then return to the center.

Repeat the pose with your left leg crossed over your right thigh. With your right hand on your left thigh, reach behind you with your left hand, gently twisting around to the left. Breathe easily for a few cycles before returning to the center.

5. **The Arch.** Place both your hands behind you, grasping the

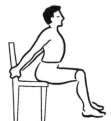

back of the chair with your hands. Inhaling slowly and deeply, lift your chest up toward the ceiling, very gently extending your neck. The stretch should be from the lower back up through the neck. Hold this posture for two deep breaths; then return to a relaxed sitting position with the next exhalation. Repeat this procedure three times.

6. **Knee Stretch.** Grasp below your right knee with both hands.

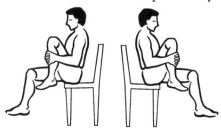

On your next inhalation, pull your knee up to your chest, feeling the stretch in your hip. On inhalation, relax and extend your thigh, gently stretching your shoulders. Perform this procedure several times on one side; then repeat it clasping your left knee with both hands.

7. **Centering Pose.** Sit quietly with your eyes closed, simply feeling the sensations in your body. Breathe easily, noticing the energy flowing within you. Enjoy the sensations that this gentle stretching has evoked.

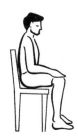

There is an expression in the Bhagavad Gita, one of the pillars of Vedic literature, that reveals the secret to a life of bliss. The Sanskrit phrase "Yogastah kuru karmani" can be translated as "Established in a state of mind-body-spirit union, perform action." In the midst of dynamic activity, we have ability to maintain our awareness in a settled state. In this state of inner quietness in the midst of action, we stay centered, regardless of the turbulence around us. The practice of yoga postures can be seen as a dynamic rehearsal for maintaining quiet inner awareness amid the challenges of modern life. This is the key to living a life rich with vital energy.

Making Vital Energy Real

Vital Stretching

1. Practice a set of yoga postures with full awareness in your body. Use your breath to enhance the connection between your mind and body. Focus your attention on the sensations in your body, rather than on achieving a final position.
2. Feel the shift in your energy before and after you stretch your body. Try performing a set of postures a few times during the day while working at your desk, flying in a plane, or riding in a car. Tune in to your body, and keep your energy moving.

Get Up and Move

Our bodies are designed for movement. Over most of the past 100,000 years that human beings have inhabited this planet, we maintained a moderately high level of physical activity. It is only in the past half century that a large proportion of our population has spent the vast majority of their days in sedentary occupations. Although I am frequently asked, "What does Ayurveda say about exercise?" I suspect that five thousand years ago the great Vedic sages did not imagine that there would be a time when human beings got into self-powered vehicles, drove fifteen minutes to the local fitness club, spent the next thirty minutes on a treadmill, then drove back home to shower before starting their workday. I remember a song from the sixties, "In the Year 2525," in which through evolution we eventually lost our bodies because we developed technology to do everything for us. Hopefully, this is not the direction nature has in mind for us, but for many people, having a body is a gift that is not fully appreciated until it begins to break down. To keep your physical vehicle running in peak condition for as long as possible, you need to exercise it regularly.

Physical exercise does not need to be complicated, but it does need to be consistent. Walking, riding a bicycle, hiking, running up stairs, Rollerblading, swimming, and dancing are as health promoting as spinning, working out on a rowing machine, or walking on a treadmill. The secret is to find some physical activity you like to do and make a commitment to do it regularly.

The Benefits of Exercise

Improved flexibility, strength, and endurance are the advantages of balanced exercise. A regular physical fitness program will improve many aspects of your physical and emotional well being. Regular physical activity can help to lower blood pressure and reduce blood cholesterol. People who exercise usually find it easier to give up harmful habits like smoking and are often able to make the shift to a better diet. Exercise stimulates the release of endorphins, our body's natural pain relievers, and regular physical activity has been shown to improve the mood in people who are depressed. Regardless of a person's physical condition or age, an appropriate exercise program can have important health benefits.

What Kind? How Much? How Often?

The most important point regarding exercise is that it be suitable for your nature. A fitness program that is right for one person may be potentially harmful to another. Your mind body type, general health, cardiac health status, beginning level of fitness, and age are all important factors in determining the optimal exercise regimen for you. Exercise should be enjoyable, and this means it needs to be appropriate for your needs.

Mind Body Type-Specific Exercise

Earth moves more slowly than the other elements, so if it predominates in your mind body constitution, you may find it difficult to find the motivation to exercise. Without regular activity, Earth becomes denser. Recent studies have suggested that people who gain weight perform fewer energy-consuming movements even at rest. Particularly if you are trying to shed a few pounds, regular physical activity is the best way to get your energy moving. If you have not been exercising for a while, start with brisk walking. In order to feel noticeable improvement in your sense of vitality, you will need to experience some sweating with your exercise, so I recommend that Earth types wear a two-layer exercise outfit. First put on a good-quality, all-cotton sweat suit, over which you can wear a nylon suit. If the weather is cool, also wear a hat. If you walk briskly with this garb, you will begin to perspire. Begin with about a half-hour of vigorous walking, gradually increasing your time. Once you begin to experience the benefits of walking, you can increase your exercise intensity to include jogging, hiking, and bicycling. If you are in reasonably good shape, playing competitive sports like basketball and soccer is a great way to work up a sweat.

Fire types need an outlet for their competitive nature, but need to be careful to not increase their stress while exercising. Swimming is probably the ideal exercise if you are a Fire type, as the water helps dissipate the heat while you are performing your laps. Long-distance bike riding, hiking, and Rollerblading are also beneficial Fire exercises. I encourage Fire people to perform their workouts outdoors whenever possible so they can bring their attention into the environment and at least temporarily out of their heated minds. Because Fire types like to compete, tennis, racquetball, and basketball are acceptable exercises, but a vigorous game should be followed by some independently performed activity like swimming to cool off both body and mind before resuming work.

Getting Wind types to exercise regularly is a challenge. They usually do not have a problem with weight control, which reduces their motivation. Their general lack of concern with routine often means a Wind person starts an exercise program, stays with it intensively for a week or two, misses one session, and then drops the intention altogether. Still, regular light exercise can help ground the agitated Wind and keep the energy moving in evolutionary directions. Exercises beneficial for Wind types focus on balance and grounding. They are generally lighter than for the other types and may include easy walking, yoga, bicycling, and dance, and their primary effects are to increase agility, coordination, and strength.

Occasionally, people who have had a Wind mind body constitution all their lives begin to gain weight excessively and appear to shift to an Earth body. This can happen after a woman gives birth and cannot lose the weight she accumulated during pregnancy. It can occur after a major illness or an overwhelming emotional challenge. The Ayurvedic explanation for this situation, when the mind is windy but the body is accumulating Earth, is that the body is attempting to ground the physiology to compensate for the uncontrollable mental turbulence. If you identify with this situation, you need to quiet your mind with meditation and then follow an Earth-reducing program for your body. A daily exercise routine is essential to reestablish balance and get your vital energy moving again in a healthy pattern. Although I am not normally a fan of exercise equipment, if you cannot perform your physical activity outdoors, a treadmill, exercise bike, rowing machine, or stair-climbing equipment can be perfect for someone with a windy mind and earthy body. The ritual, rhythmic workout performed with music that has a good beat can help restore balance to both the Wind and Earth elements.

Choosing the appropriate exercise for your body type ensures the most benefit and the greatest enjoyment. If you are performing some physical activity for the sake of your health but are finding it a strain, it will not provide the benefit you are seeking, and you will probably not stay with it for very long. The body is designed to move and thrives on regular activity. Regardless of your current state of physical fitness, moving helps vital energy to flow.

Recovering Fitness

If you have a history of heart disease or have not been physically active for some time, your exercise prescription should be designed in conjunction with your physician and exercise physiologist. I recommend that you approach improving your general and cardiac fitness in stages.

Stage 1 Stretching

The initial goal is to develop comfortable body movements. Begin with a basic set of yoga postures designed to create flexibility with a focus on integrating your breathing with the positions. These poses should be performed with sensitivity to your level of comfort. Straining is contrary to the very nature of yoga. If you have been recovering from an illness, suffer with chronic pain, or are severely overweight, gently stretching with awareness is the first step to reconnecting your body and mind.

Stage 2 Moving with Awareness

As you become comfortable with the flexibility postures, progressing to more active movements can enhance your circulatory function. Maintaining awareness of your internal bodily signals remains essential at this stage. It is useful to take your pulse at rest and during and at the end of activity. If you are basically healthy, I recommend gradually increasing your exercise level so that your heart rate rises no more than 50 percent from baseline during the first month. For example, if your resting heart rate is 80 beats per minute, your pulse should stay below 120 beats per minute.

A set of yoga postures called the Sun Salutations provides an excellent balanced exercise to improve flexibility. This is a series of twelve yoga postures that can be performed vigorously to increase your heart rate. You can pace the rate and number of sets that are performed to meet your target heart rate. Walking, light swimming, and bicycling are also appropriate for this stage.

SUN SALUTATIONS

The twelve positions of the Sun Salutations can be performed slowly or briskly. Earth types—perform rapidly; Fire types—perform at a medium pace; and Wind types—perform steadily. Pictured on page 174, the Sun Salutations provide an ideal training program as they stretch and tone all parts of the body.

1. Salutation pose: Begin with your palms together in front of your chest, breathing easily.
2. Raised-arms pose: Stretch upward and extend toward the sky with your head between your arms.
3. Hand-to-foot pose: Gently bending from the hips, bring your hands toward your feet.
4. Equestrian pose: Slide your left leg back as you lower the left knee and both hands to the ground. Look up.
5. Mountain pose: Bring your right leg backward, even with the left. Raise your buttocks, look down at your feet, and gently lower your heels to the ground.
6. Eight limbs pose: Lower your knees, chest, and chin to the ground, keeping your buttocks lightly raised.
7. Cobra pose: Lower your pelvis down. Raise your forehead, chin, and chest, lifting primarily with your abdominal muscles, not your arms.
8. Mountain pose: You are now reversing the order of the positions, rising back into the mountain pose.
9. Equestrian pose: Again slide your leg back as you lower your right knee and both hands to the ground.
10. Hand-to-foot pose: Bring your leg forward, even with the other side, bending at the waist.
11. Raised-arms pose: Stretch your arms upward as you inhale.
12. Salutation pose: Return to the resting position with both palms together in front of your chest.

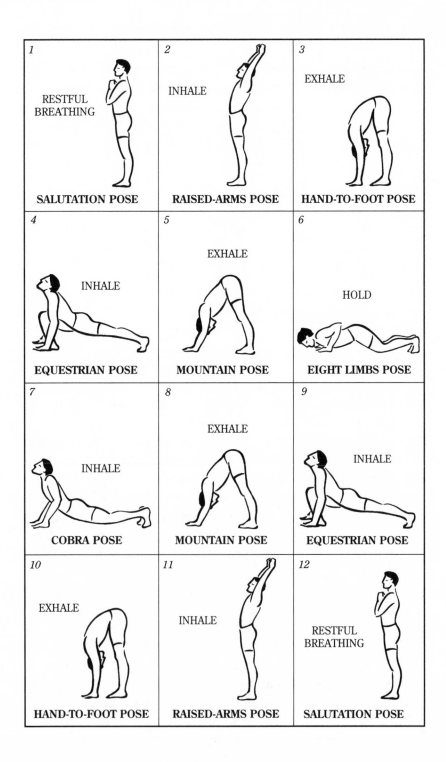

1	2	3
RESTFUL BREATHING **SALUTATION POSE**	INHALE **RAISED-ARMS POSE**	EXHALE **HAND-TO-FOOT POSE**

4	5	6
INHALE **EQUESTRIAN POSE**	EXHALE **MOUNTAIN POSE**	HOLD **EIGHT LIMBS POSE**

7	8	9
INHALE **COBRA POSE**	EXHALE **MOUNTAIN POSE**	INHALE **EQUESTRIAN POSE**

10	11	12
EXHALE **HAND-TO-FOOT POSE**	INHALE **RAISED-ARMS POSE**	RESTFUL BREATHING **SALUTATION POSE**

174

Maintain full awareness in your body while you are performing these poses. Perform between two and twenty cycles per session.

Stage 3 Building Fitness

If you are feeling comfortable with the flexibility and light aerobic exercises in Stages 1 and 2, you may gradually increase the intensity of your aerobic activity to meet the recommended target zone for your age. The same activities performed during Stage 2 can be increased in time and intensity, including the Sun Salutations, brisk walking, swimming, and bicycling. Jogging and dancing may also be appropriate.

In general I suggest that you aim for a training heart rate of 80 percent of maximal with a range from 60 to 90 percent. To calculate this number:

1. Subtract your age from 220.
2. Multiply this number by .80.

For example, if you are 45 years old, your target heart rate during exercise is calculated as the following:

1. $220 - 45 = 175$
2. $175 \times .80 = 140$ beats per minute

For most people, an exercise program that reaches the target heart rate provides optimal fitness benefit when performed for twenty to thirty minutes, three times per week.

In addition, keep in mind the following points:

- During peak exercise, you should have a thin film of perspiration, but you should not be sweating profusely, as this may mean your body is becoming overheated.
- You should be able to hold a light conversation while you are exercising. If you are unable to talk at all because you are short of breath, you should reduce the intensity of your workout.
- Above all, emphasize exercises that you truly enjoy.
- Each exercise session should include a warm-up stretching period, an active phase, and a cooling-down phase.

An ideal fifty-minute fitness session might include the following:

1. Ten minutes of meditation
2. Ten minutes of yoga postures with breathing awareness
3. Twenty minutes of aerobic activity
4. Five minutes of yoga postures
5. Five minutes of quiet resting

The yoga component provides flexibility and strength, and the aerobic exercise provides the endurance training. If done with family, friends, or classmates to great music, it should be fun as well as beneficial to your health.

Exercise Precautions

The following precautions are recommended to maximize the benefits and minimize any risks associated with a cardiovascular fitness program:

- Wait at least ninety minutes after a meal before exercising.
- Do not exercise when you are not feeling well (with a cold, flu, or viral illness) as your body needs rest, not exertion, when it is facing an illness.
- Discontinue exercising if you have chest discomfort, palpitations, or dizziness, and promptly notify your physician.
- Warm up and cool down gradually; do not engage in sudden vigorous physical activity.

Increase your activity gradually over time to develop aerobic endurance. Be sensitive to your internal signals of comfort while paying attention to your breathing pattern and pulse. At the Chopra Center we recommend chest-worn heart rate monitors that transmit information to a wrist receiver as a means of amplifying the feedback loop between heart and mind. These electronic feedback systems allow you to continuously observe your heartbeat and assess both subjectively and objectively the level of exercise intensity that is best for you.

There are lots of reasons why today is not the right day to start exercising. None of them are valid. Put this book down right now and go for a brisk walk! Your body, mind, and spirit will thank you.

Making Vital Energy Real

Vital Movement

1. Begin a physical activity program today. Check your pulse at rest, and (assuming you do not have a history of heart disease) do something active to get your heart beating faster and harder.
2. Commit to a regular exercise program that includes stretching and aerobic activity at least three times per week for twenty to thirty minutes.
3. Over the course of several weeks, gradually increase your activity intensity until you are able to reach 75 to 80 percent of your maximum heart rate. Notice how quickly your endurance and your vitality improve.

Get Stronger

Give me three minutes of your time. Get out a wristwatch with a second hand and take the following muscular fitness test. It is designed to both evaluate your current strength status and demonstrate how easy it is to begin a strength-enhancing program.

1. Drop prone to the floor and see how many push-ups you can do over the next thirty seconds. If you can only perform a few before your arms tire out, rest a few moments and try again before the thirty seconds are up. If you cannot perform even one push-up with your full body weight, then try doing them on your knees. When the thirty seconds are up, rest for the next half-minute; then turn onto your back.
2. With your knees bent and your hands behind your head, perform abdominal crunches for the next thirty seconds. The de-

sired movement is just enough to raise your upper body off the floor. See how many you can do in half a minute. When the time is up, rest for a few moments, then stand up.

3. See how many deep knee bends you can do in thirty seconds. Squat down until your knees are at a ninety-degree angle while keeping your back straight and perpendicular to the floor. If you have had an injury to your knees, perform this exercise very carefully. Rest after doing these knee bends for a half-minute.

You have now completed a three-minute strength-building exercise program. To whatever degree you were able to perform these exercises, you now have a platform to build upon. See where you rank on the following scale.

	Push-ups	Ab Crunches	Knee Bends
Tender	fewer than 10	fewer than 10	fewer than 10
Promising	10–19	10–19	10–19
Recovering	20–29	20–29	20–29
Pumped!	30 or more	30 or more	30 or more

Spend three minutes three times a day, and within a very short time you will find yourself gaining in strength and muscle tone. If you want to add other exercises, you can position a pull-up bar in a doorway to exercise your biceps. You can use free weights or ankle weights to isolate specific arm or leg muscles. You do not need to join a fitness gym or purchase expensive workout equipment to build muscle fitness, and so you have no excuse not to spend ten minutes a day improving your strength.

Sitting in an office chair for eight hours a day, driving a car, and lounging on the sofa in front of the television are the standard of physical activity for many North Americans. Not only are adults guilty of a drift toward increasingly sedentary lifestyles, but our children are also doing less physical activity and showing increasing trends toward health-damaging obesity. It doesn't take a tremendous amount of time to improve our physical fitness. It does require some attention and a modicum of discipline. The payoff is worth it on many levels.

Making Vital Energy Real

Enhance Your Strength

1. Begin a muscular fitness program today.
2. If you wish to join a fitness club or purchase home workout equipment, great, but don't use the absence of a facility or exercise machines to justify delaying or avoiding a regular strength-enhancing program.
3. Try the three-minute workouts three times daily for one week and discover how quickly and easily you can tone your body.

Honor Your Body

I have seen many spiritually minded people who, believing that their souls inhabit, but are transcendent to, their bodies, neglect their bodies in favor of their spiritual side. Not until their bodies become weak or ill do they receive the attention they deserve. Many people I see each day in my practice take better care of their automobiles than their bodies (and most do not take great care of their cars). We assume responsibility for a remarkable living vehicle at the time of our birth, and the better we care for it, the better it will serve our needs without causing discomfort or distress. You don't have to spend hours in a gym every day to maintain physical fitness. Ten minutes of yoga, twenty minutes of aerobic activity, and five minutes of toning exercises five days a week will accomplish the goal of creating a healthy and fit body. The same creative force that generated the universe created your body. It is vibrating with intelligence and spirit. It is ultimately sacred and worthy of your respect, love, and attention. Take good care of it and it will take good care of you.

Vital Energy Key #6

Work with Meaning,
Play with Passion

I am water rushing to the well-head
filling the pitcher until it spills. —JANE KENYON

Why are we here? Almost every individual, every society, and
every spiritual tradition has asked this question. Freud said we're
here to love and to work. Mother Teresa inspired us to serve in
God's name. Hindus strive for enlightenment. Buddhists seek
Nirvana. Christians aim to do Christ's work on earth. Jews seek
the Messianic age. The answers we choose from the marketplace
of salvation set the trajectory for our life's journey. Regardless of
the ultimate goal you see for your duration on this planet, one
thing is true. We are here for a short time, and finding meaning
and purpose in our daily activity is essential if we are to experience
vitality in our lives.

A consistent theme in every spiritual tradition is the belief that
we are in this world but not of this world. I experience pleasure

and pain, loss and gain, but the real me is beyond the ups and downs of time-bound awareness. This is the great paradox of being human. We are simultaneously unbounded beings of spirit—drops of light in the vast ocean of universal light—and localized, ego-based individuals, concerned about making car payments, wearing a flattering hairstyle, and finding a good Italian restaurant. Unless you have chosen a monastic life, you have to function in the world. The key to vital living is making choices that are most likely to bring joy and passion into your life. A life with richness and meaning is a vital life. Let's explore some of the ingredients of enthusiastic living.

Find Your Dharma

What do you want to be when you grow up? Most of us were asked this question from an early age by family members and friends. As a child you may have gone through a phase of wanting to be a teacher, a fireman, an actor, a veterinarian, or a baseball player. In spite of our efforts to avoid gender stereotyping, families and society provide powerful reinforcements for vocational choices. As children we try on different roles and witness the responses to our choice of the day from those whose approval we seek. If you were raised in a blue-collar family in the Midwest, announcing that you wanted to be an artist may not have received the most positive encouragement from your parents. Announcing to your family of bankers that you were thinking of devoting your life to nursing might have met with a similar lack of enthusiasm. In my family I got the message that a fetus became a human being on the day it graduated from medical school. Some of these guiding influences are subtle and some not, but they do provide value. Parents want their children to have more comfortable, happier lives, and it is their legitimate role to guide their offspring in pursuit of this goal. On the other hand, each of us has unique talents that we long to express, and children are not mere lumps of clay waiting to be molded by society. Ultimately, it is the role of parents to help their children discover what it is that they can do well and with enthusiasm.

Ayurveda offers the beautiful concept of dharma. Often translated as "the way," dharma suggests that each of us traverses a path through life that provides us with the experiences we need to gain wisdom. When we are consciously on the path of dharma, life becomes magical. Each event has meaning, and circumstances seem to defy the laws of probability. The phone rings a moment after we think of someone we want to speak with, we run into old friends in foreign cities, and the page of the book we open to just happens to address the concern we've been contemplating. We have an underlying sense that there is intelligence in the universe and that we have the password to the cosmic Web site. As adults, dharma implies that we are enthusiastic about the work we are doing, which provides satisfaction and fulfillment to ourselves and all those affected by our labors.

How do we find our dharma? Most of us did not arrive with instructions that spelled out what we should be doing with our lives. Modern educational systems are less concerned with each of us finding our place than with our finding any place that can keep the wheels of the economy turning. The wisdom of dharma comes from within and is best accessed by listening to your quiet inner voice. Use the following exercises to assess where you are and where you'd like to be.

WORK SATISFACTION QUESTIONNAIRE

1. How satisfied am I with my current work?

Please respond to the following questions as honestly and accurately as possible.

	Characteristic of me . . .				
	Not at all	*Slightly*	*Somewhat*	*Moderately*	*Very*
1. I look forward to going in to work on Monday morning.	1	2	3	4	5

	Characteristic of me …				
	Not at all	*Slightly*	*Somewhat*	*Moderately*	*Very*
2. I consider several of my coworkers to be good friends.	1	2	3	4	5
3. I am able to express my creativity in my work.	1	2	3	4	5
4. I often find myself losing track of time at work.	1	2	3	4	5
5. I feel appreciated at work.	1	2	3	4	5

Work satisfaction score: _____

Scoring:

9 or less   Work is a real drudgery for you. If you are not now ill, continuing to work in your current environment will lead to emotional or physical distress.

10 to 15   Work is providing marginal benefit for you. You are probably bored most of the time and perceive little opportunity for improvement.

16 to 20   Work can be a source of nourishment for you. With some conscious attention, the work you are doing may blossom into your dharma.

21 to 25   You are in your dharma. The boundaries between your life and your work are fluid. Your main challenge is to balance your work needs with those of your family.

2. What do I want to be when I grow up?

(If you scored 21 or more points on part 1, you can skip this part.)

Answer the following questions as honestly as possible.

1. What do I do well?

_____

_____

_____

2. What work do I dream about doing that I can enjoy?

_____

_____

_____

3. What will it take to make the transition from my current work to work that is meaningful for me?

_____

_____

_____

How do you know when you are in your dharma? When you are living your dharma, you do not think about what you'd rather be doing. Time loses its grip as you become absorbed in the present moment. You feel that you are made to do what you are doing and that the universe was made to provide you the opportunity to express your talents. Energy flows without resistance. Living in dharma allows the expression of selfless selfishness. You are doing exactly what you find most nourishing and at the same time providing value to everyone affected by your actions.

A vital life is one in which nourishment predominates and toxicity is minimized. Considering that many of us spend close to one-third of our lives on the job, it is not surprising that our mental and physical well being can be influenced by how happy or miserable we are while working. Look at your workplace as you look at your home. How can you change the sensations in your surroundings from toxic to nourishing? The same work performed in an environment where the sounds, sights, and smells are uplifting can be much more gratifying than when performed in a less nurturing space.

Heal the relationships with your coworkers. We can create heaven or hell through our relations with others. Regardless of the history up until now, you have the opportunity to change things if you choose to see those around you as your mirrors. Try something different. Invite your petty tyrant at work to lunch and find out what makes that person tick. Sit down with a troublesome boss or employee and see if you can connect on a person-to-person level rather than jousting role to role. A person living in dharma carries no resentments, does not need another's approval, and does not seek to control others. Whether or not you are living your dream work, you can use your current enterprise to practice living dharmically. Begin taking steps in the direction of what you really want to do and heed the feedback from your soul via your body. Unbounded vitality is a side benefit of living in dharma.

Work for Your Mind Body Type

I believe that employment agencies would have an easier time placing people into the right jobs if they considered their mind body constitutions. We assess people's natures unconsciously whenever we are considering someone for a role in an organization. We are unlikely to hire a thin, delicate Wind type to be a piano mover and would not choose a shy, quiet being to host a lively television game show. Depending upon your mind body nature, you may be better suited to one kind of work than to another.

Earth Work

Society and organizations are built on the foundation of Earth beings, for they provide the solid consistency that supports institutions at their base. Earth types enjoy routine and usually thrive in roles that allow them to provide stability and nurturing. Earth types make good managers, as the hassles inherent in organizations do not easily ruffle them. The best administrators in every organization have the right balance of a solid Earth energy with just enough Fire to lead and Wind to inspire their team members. Too much Fire, and managers become domineering and lose the trust of their staff. Too much Wind, and they have difficulty keeping their work priorities separate from their personal issues. Earth people are comfortable assuming responsibility that engenders loyalty.

Professional caregivers, including nurses, therapists, and social workers, often have a predominance of Earth in their nature. Earth people enjoy acting as teachers and coaches, receiving satisfaction in the accomplishments of those they've guided. The risk for Earth types is getting stuck in a role that is too routine and mundane, leading to stagnation and congestion. When their vital energy is flowing, Earth people provide the structure of an organization, but if they are stagnating, they become calcified and bureaucratic. If your nature is predominantly Earth, try consciously adding some variety to your daily routine to culture flexibility. Drive to work by a different route, wear clothing outside your usual style, and make it a point to talk to a coworker in a way that expresses more than the usual platitudes. Recognize how people around you instantly notice even subtle changes in your routine, commenting on the new dress or sweater you are wearing, your different hairstyle, or your shift toward a more open communication style. Let the earth move, and energizing vital energy will become available to you.

Fire Work

People who have a predominance of Fire in their systems do their best work when precision and attention to detail are important. Fire people thrive as engineers, computer programmers, accountants, and editors. They need a sense of completion at the end of the day and do not tolerate ambiguity well. An ongoing concern for Fire types is getting squeezed by time constraints. Those with an abundance of heat in their system do not like to see work that has not been carefully reviewed. Minor errors become sources of irritation and a deadline fans the flames of aggravation. When Fire types are balanced, they can be good managers, but when they are feeling overloaded, they can be intimidating and abrasive. If you have a preponderance of Fire in your nature, you will be happiest if you set realistic goals for yourself with a good balance of work and play.

If I had to reduce the internal conversation of Fire to a single word, it would be "more." This is the nature of the metabolism element that is continually seeking new fuel to combust. As long as the transformational process is in balance, energy is made available and the fire burns cleanly. Fire types need to be vigilant to not let their desires consume their resources, resulting in depletion. Regardless of the occupational role Fire people play, when they hear their inner dialogue heating up, they need to cool off. Excessive thoughts about not getting enough recognition, feeling unsupported, or comparing yourself to others are clues that you need to take some cooling, deep breaths or a few days off to reset your balance point. Pay attention to the early signs of a Fire imbalance and you will avoid burnout.

Wind Work

If Wind is the predominant force in your constitution, you will feel most harmonious with work that allows you flexibility. You will not thrive in a job that is inherently routine. While your Earth friends may do fine working on a computer assembly line and your Fire colleagues may enjoy generating detailed financial statements, you will quickly get bored in a job that is repetitive or too detail-oriented. This is despite the fact that some work routine can be good for Wind types, providing a stabilizing rhythm.

Sales, marketing, and public relations may be ideal positions for Wind types, who thrive on communication and change. These roles allow for a considerable degree of autonomy and draw upon personality style as much as learned skills. Public speaking, entertainment, and politics can offer great opportunities for Wind beings to express their energy and creativity. When there is ample opportunity for innovation, teaching can be a good role for a Wind person. If you remember back to your elementary school days, some of your best teachers were probably lively and enthusiastic Wind types. Unfortunately, most school curriculums do not tolerate much originality, and our entertaining Wind teachers often move on to other roles where their creative energies are more appreciated. The consistent Earth teachers and disciplined Fire instructors tend to be the ones who stay in teaching for the long run.

Those with Wind in their sails do not thrive if their day offers no surprises. They need novelty and challenge to prosper. Of course the challenge is to balance the need for originality with a rhythm that supports recentering. A Wind type is easily swept up in the enthusiasm of the project, neglects the basics of eating well and getting enough rest, and gets off balance. People with Wind in their natures must integrate enough routine in their days to balance their high-energy tendencies. They require grounding to maintain their equilibrium.

Regardless of your predominant mind body nature, create work that you can perform with passion. When you are expending energy in an activity that brings you joy and satisfaction, vital energy flows through every cell in your body. The well of vitality is inexhaustible when you are performing dharmic work in service to yourself and others.

Making Vital Energy Real

Discover Your Purpose

1. Create work that nourishes your body, mind, and soul. Do not tolerate a toxic working environment.
2. Begin with the recognition that you have unique qualities and talents that can be expressed in your work. If it is not the time to make a big change, try taking small steps in the direction of fulfilling your dharma.
3. Ask yourself the important questions—How can I be of service? How can I help? What am I here to bring to the world? Listen to the messages that arise, and follow your heart.

Create Wealth Consciousness

Money, which represents the prose of life, and which is hardly spoken of in parlors without an apology, is, in its effects and laws, as beautiful as roses. —RALPH WALDO EMERSON

Everybody thinks about money. I recently took a survey of people at the Chopra Center for Well Being, asking the question: How many times each day do you think about money? I was surprised at the responses I received. The answers ranged from only occasionally to almost continuously, but on average, people at a center dedicated to spiritual transformation admitted that they think about money at least ten times per day. This includes everyone from the director of programming to the delivery person.

What do people think about when they think about money? Most people think about how they are going to pay for things they already have (e.g., pay off credit cards or the mortgage), how they are going to pay for things they want to have (e.g., a new car, a vacation), and how they might work less but have more. Some people spend time each day calculating how much money they currently have, comparing it to how much they believe they need if they are to have the easier life they are seeking.

Most of us are uncomfortable talking about money; it makes us feel vulnerable. Deep down, we don't really believe that a person's financial worth has any direct relationship to his or her value as a human being, but we live in a society where money buys power and opportunity. Those who have more money are concerned about being too conspicuous, and those who have less are concerned about not appearing as successful as they believe they deserve to be. With few exceptions, almost everyone dreams about having more money.

We can learn a lot from these exceptions. People who rarely think about money tend to be lighthearted beings, having relinquished the need for the approval of others. They do what brings them joy, allowing their creativity to flow. As a consequence of expressing their unique talents, they have enough money. Rather than focusing on making money so they can eventually quit doing what they have to do and start doing what they want to do, they simply choose to do what they want, now. These tend to be among the most creative people in the world, for they do not squander their energy worrying about the future.

You may be thinking that this level of freedom sounds wonderful, but considering the car payment, mortgage, credit card debt, and the children's school tuition that face you, it will not be your experience in this lifetime. As is true with almost every aspect of life on this planet of opposites, the secret to vital living is to find balance in the midst of polarity. This means you do not have to sell the house and move to Costa Rica to have a less pressured life. You do need to honestly assess your current lifestyle and decide whether more will necessarily mean better. At almost every economic stratum, you can find people living more simply, which means that if you choose, you can as well. To move in the direction of greater financial balance, you will need to listen to your quiet inner voice, rather than the clamor to buy more that surrounds us. To get in touch with your relationship to money, ask yourself the following questions:

1. How much stress am I currently experiencing over money issues?
2. How much of my current stress is due to actual financial concerns versus not having as much money as I would like?
3. How much money do I actually need to cover my necessities in life?
4. In what ways might I be able to simplify my life so I am not consumed by the need to earn money?
5. Are there activities I would choose to engage in (classes at a local college, music lessons, hiking, etc.) if I were not so focused on making money?

How much is enough? For some of my patients, even a net worth of tens of millions of dollars is not enough because they measure their value in comparison to others who possess more. Every fluctuation in the stock market generates exhilaration or despair. On the other hand, I see people of modest means who are living rich and abundant lives. Reality is always a selective act of perception and interpretation, and we have the power to choose a reality that can make us happy or miserable. Listen to your body for messages of comfort and discomfort. If worries over maintaining your lifestyle are keeping you up at night, giving you an ulcer, raising your blood pressure, or exhausting you, *it isn't worth it.* Stop comparing yourself to others. Rather, find the financial perspective that will satisfy you without making yourself or those around you sick.

Mind Body and Money

Your relationship to money will be influenced by your mind body constitution. If Wind is the most predominant element in your nature, your tendency will be to spend what you have, without a consistent concern to save for the future. You like money for the freedom it offers and tend to spend impulsively. If you unexpectedly receive a small inheritance or tax refund, you are likely to go on a shopping spree, choosing items that appeal to you without much deliberation. Your challenge is to acknowledge your natural impulsivity and consciously create some financial discipline. Be careful about choosing investments that are too speculative. Try allocating a portion of your income for savings in investment vehicles that do not allow you to withdraw your money the moment you fall in love with a new car or piece of jewelry.

If the Fire element dominates your nature, your relationship with money will tend to be around issues of control. You closely identify the expenditure of your life energy with the money you make and have and are not comfortable relinquishing control to a partner, spouse, or financial consultant. When you spend money, it is usually for things that enhance your status such as nice cars, houses, paintings, or jewelry. You usually like to do your homework before making purchases and may spend a disproportionate amount of time analyzing a deal compared to the amount of money you actually save. In order to create a healthy relationship with money, Fire types need to allocate some portion of their income purely for enjoyment. This means accepting that it is okay to occasionally be frivolous and enjoy the experience of letting go. Fire types also benefit from learning to be generous and charitable. One of the best things a person with Fire can do to improve his or her vital energy is to give something away anonymously. In so doing, you can learn the value of allowing your heart to flow without directly receiving compensation for your actions. Learning to trust the cosmic accounting system will reduce the energy wasted on trying to control life too closely.

The earth is composed of water and land, and if the Earth element is predominant in your nature, your relationship to money may have contrasting qualities. On one hand, you like to spend money on sensual pleasures—delicious meals, luxurious massages, exotic colognes. On the other hand, Earth types have a hibernation impulse that at times leads to a hoarding mentality. If this is in your nature, you may find it difficult to spend money, or even to invest. Extreme Earth types tend to find comfort in doomsday scenarios in which the entire world economy collapses and their gold coins stashed under the mattress are the only way for them to survive. If you have a dominance of Earth in your constitution, think in terms of circulation. If you are financially constipated, practice allowing some of the energy you are storing in the form of money to flow and notice the sense of freedom and vitality that follows.

Abundance Consciousness

Abundance consciousness is a state of awareness in which our happiness is independent of our possessions and positions in life. To the extent we have established direct access to our inner reservoir of energy and creativity, we have wealth consciousness. How do we generate this state? By honoring the affluence of nature as she expresses itself through our unique mind body constitution. This means tapping into our reservoir of abundance through inner exploration and through expression of our innate talents in the world. Find what it is that allows you to do well and to do good. Express yourself in work that enables your juices to flow and provides nourishment to you and all those touched by your work. Time stands still when you are doing exactly what you were made to do, and material, emotional, and spiritual abundance flow through you. Relinquish the idea that you will be happy or feel safe once you have a certain amount of money in the bank. Create wealth, but don't mistake the experience of abundance for the objects of affluence. Enjoy what you have, create what you want, and never lose a sense of connection to your inner reservoir of energy and creativity.

Making Vital Energy Real

Vital Abundance

1. Organize your life so you are not depleting your vital energy worrying about money. Simplify your lifestyle to a point that allows you some degree of financial freedom and frees up your creativity to generate abundance in your life.
2. Honestly assess what you want and what you need. Realize that with ownership comes responsibility. Ultimately, things own us as much as we own them.
3. Understand how you intrinsically relate to money and strive for a balance between enjoying the present moment and preparing for the future. Remember that "enough" is a state of awareness rather than a specific number.

Enjoy Your Friends

Friendship is Love without his wings. —LORD BYRON

Despite the fact that more people are living on the planet than ever before, each day I see my patients living alienated and lonely lives. Almost without exception, I find myself feeling tremendous compassion and love for these lonely souls who on some level believe they are unlovable. Sometimes this takes the form of self-recrimination; other times it manifests as disdain for others, as in "Everyone I work with cares about superficial things," or "My roommate is so self-absorbed, all she talks about is herself." In either case, the artificial boundaries between self and others build a wall that effectively limits the flow of vital energy to nourish body, mind, and soul. Like a body of water that does not flow, stagnation leads to toxicity.

What is the basis of a nurturing friendship? The answer is in being able to see the unity beyond the diversity. A woman I saw recently in consultation described the reason for her breakups with each past lover: "I realized we were two completely different people!" Although it is nice to imagine that somewhere on this planet there is someone who has all the same opinions, interests, likes, and dislikes you have, you will almost certainly spend many lonely years waiting for that person. Ultimately we make a choice to focus on those aspects that unite us with, or separate us from, others.

How do we create relationships that serve their highest purpose of reminding us of our universal nature? Like everything in life, that which we put our attention on grows stronger. To create nurturing friendships we need to work on giving what we want for ourselves. Five basic components of a supportive, nurturing relationship must be present for each person to feel satisfied. We can remember these aspects by the mnemonic *ADORE*, which stands for *A*ccept, *D*emonstrate, *O*pen, *R*eceive, and *E*xpress. Let's take them one at a time.

Accept Yourself, Accept Others

Acceptance allows us to be ourselves in the presence of others. Hopefully, you had a taste of unconditional acceptance as a baby when your parents relished every movement, facial expression, and sound that emerged from you. Unfortunately, most relationships are based on needs and expectations, rather than acceptance. We give and receive strong messages that if approval, attention, or appreciation are to be granted, you must be or act in a specific way that is deemed acceptable. Like Zelig, the chameleon-like character in Woody Allen's movie, many of us spend our lives trying to change into a form we believe others will appreciate.

True friendship results from the recognition that there is more than one way to live a life, and that our differences are the basis of passion. As we explored in chapter 4, each of us has many facets to our personality and plays many different roles each day. I have serious and silly sides, mature and childish aspects, wise and foolish parts in my nature. The more I can own all these flavors in my personality, the more easily I can accept these qualities in you. Ultimately, acceptance of others is a reflection of the extent to which we are able to accept ourselves. When the voice of judgment and comparison is shouting loudly in your head, ask what the voice is saying about you as much as about the person you are judging. Understand and embrace the many facets of your nature, and you will find your ability to accept others growing spontaneously in your life.

Demonstrate Your Caring

How do people know you care about them? How do you know people care about you? The answer is through our words and deeds. We need to demonstrate our caring, appreciation, and concern for the people in our lives since most of us have not mastered mental telepathy. Small gestures—an unexpected phone call, a friendly note, a bouquet of flowers, a neck massage, baking cookies—can carry as much weight as big ones. Actively demonstrate your appreciation for your close friends and family with physical affection. Animals need caressing, babies thrive on massage, and adult human beings flourish when they are lovingly touched. A neck rub, a shoulder massage, and a warm hug can be nourishing to mind and body. Loving touch can lower blood pressure, reduce pain, and enhance immunity. Demonstrate your willingness to be intimate by touching the people you love sensitively and often.

Open Your Heart

The only way to obtain nourishment from the environment is to let it in. Maintaining the right balance between openness and safety is the major challenge for human beings in relationships. You can have your defenses on high alert and not allow anyone into your place of vulnerability. You may avoid being hurt, but then you will definitely avoid being loved. On the other end of the spectrum, you can open your heart without discernment and find your tender places being trounced. The basic message is: find the right balance.

Risk is a part of life—without a willingness to try something new you cannot experience any reality other than the one familiar to you. If you are overflowing in vitality, love, creativity, and enthusiasm, keep doing what you are doing. If you are craving something more on a physical, emotional, or spiritual level, you need to open to uncertainty. Urban dwellers take hikes in the woods because we enjoy the uncertainty that comes with unfamiliar terrain. Hiking in the wilderness opens the possibility for encountering something unexpected as well as getting lost. Cultivating flexibility allows you to bend more easily without breaking to life's inevitable challenges.

We keep our emotional guard up because we have been hurt in the past. To get beyond the limitations imposed by the fear of opening, you will need to embrace and release your pain and start choosing people who tread gently in your inner sanctum. As you develop your comfort level with the light and dark sides of your being, you will attract people into your life who support your expanding wholeness, rather than those who zap your energy.

Receive Love

There is really little difference between giving and receiving. When you give something of yourself to people who openly receive it, expressing and demonstrating their appreciation for your effort, who gets the benefit? The beauty of giving is that the giver always receives and the receiver always gives. I see many people in my practice, usually women, who spend their entire lives nurturing others, viewing themselves as "givers." Then, when they have exhausted themselves or find themselves facing a major emotional or physical challenge, they find it difficult to ask for or receive help. They don't want to be a burden on others.

Although at times it is true that people used to receiving may not be very comfortable returning the favor, most people relish the opportunity to be of service to others. I often hear parents saying they do not want to be a burden on their children, but caring for people we love does not need to be a burden. Most parents do not think that caring for their children for eighteen-plus years is burdensome. For most of humanity's time on this planet, the social security system has consisted of extended multigenerational families. Be open to receiving the love and attention of others, knowing that in accepting their affection you are providing them something valuable in return.

One of the most powerful ways to receive is simply to listen attentively when another person is communicating. Allowing other people to express their thoughts and feelings while providing your attention is a gift that deeply nourishes. Infants and children thrive on conscious listening, for this is how we learn we are worthy of attention. Healthy relationships are based on conscious communication in which both parties are honestly expressing and listening. If you find yourself regularly cutting people off or finishing their sentences, it is a sign that you are reacting rather than responding. Practice conscious listening and see how much more effective your communication can be. If you notice other people regularly interrupting you, politely ask them to wait until you have completed your thought before responding, and commit that you will do the same. Each of us needs to be heard, which cannot occur if both people are speaking at the same time. Be open to receiving the energy of others and vitality will flow in your life.

Express Your Love

Tell the people you appreciate that you appreciate them. Tell the people you love that you love them. For example, even if your husband has been taking care of your landscaping for years, he still likes to know that his care is appreciated. Even if your wife has been balancing the checkbook for years, she still enjoys hearing her work acknowledged. Be generous with your words of praise and approval. All of us like to hear that our efforts are noticed and valued. Catch people doing things well and right and acknowledge them.

It is equally important that you be willing to express your feelings. The most likely way to get your needs met is to ask for what you want. This means learning to express your feelings in ways that make it easy for someone else to respond to you. Avoid blaming others for your feelings. Express them in a way that demonstrates that you are taking responsibility for your emotions and are committed to creating healthier communication patterns to enhance both parties' experience of the relationship. Ultimately, the quality of any relationship is based on the quality of communication. Commit to expressing yourself with honesty and openness, and your relationships will be sources of abundant vital energy.

Friends in Deed

We can choose our friends and they can choose us. Unlike family relationships, which for better or worse will be there on some level for the duration of our time here, friends come and go throughout our lives. They can be our clearest mirrors, precisely because there is an element of choice in the relationship. Cultivate your friendships so they can be sources of nurturing and vitality. Enjoy your friends. A good sign of the health of a friendship is how often you laugh together. Although you can take your friends seriously, don't let your friendships be too serious. The essence of our self, the essence of spirit, is lightheartedness. The essence of friendship is that we can be ourselves. So the essence of friendship is lightheartedness. Open your heart to your dear friends and release the heaviness that inhibits your vitality.

Making Vital Energy Real

Vital Friendship

1. Practice creating conscious friendships based upon mutual trust and respect. Make a list of those qualities you consider essential components of a nurturing friendship. Look at each component and honestly evaluate the extent to which you are able to provide those ingredients. Consider what you want in your relationships and what you are willing to invest.
2. Look at your friendships and see if there are ways you can enhance them by accepting, demonstrating, opening, receiving,

and expressing. Use your relationships as mirrors of yourself to deepen your connection to your inner reservoir of energy and vitality.

Go Outside to Play

We can never have enough of Nature. —HENRY DAVID THOREAU

Most kids like to play outdoors. There is a freedom and newness to exploring the environment that is exhilarating and rejuvenating. As adults we tend to forget the power of connecting with our natural surroundings until we feel overwhelmed by the routine of modern life and decide we have to get away to Hawaii or Costa Rica before we spontaneously combust from stress. Vacations are great and can be revitalizing, assuming you don't exhaust yourself trying to have fun. Of greater value than an occasional holiday is scheduling regular time to connect with your environment. As discussed in the first chapter, according to Ayurveda the world is composed of five major elements—space, air, fire, water, and earth. We can connect with these natural forces by focusing our attention on them. Let's explore each one in more detail.

Space Energy

Ultimately, everything in the material world can be reduced to space. Even solid objects are mostly emptiness when seen from a quantum-mechanical perspective. When we put our attention on space, we experience lightness and openness in our awareness. The most direct way to access the qualities of space in your environment is to put your attention on the sky. Find a comfortable place in a park, spread out a blanket, lie on your back, and gaze into the sky. Watch the clouds transform and dissolve and allow the deep blue openness to expand your mind. Whenever you go out at night, look up at the moon and into the stars and contemplate the relationship between your current concerns and the vastness of the cosmos. Get to know the stars. Connecting with nature by gazing into the heavens allows us to experience our unboundedness in the midst of localized individuality. Whenever you find yourself agonizing over little things, look into the enormity of the universe. It helps put life into perspective.

Air Energy

The air element represents the movement of space. Subtle yet essential to life, air is the most refined expression of matter. As living beings our most intimate experience with air is through our respiration. Breathing connects our environment, body, mind, and spirit. The molecules of oxygen we inhale arise as by-products of a green plant's alchemical conversion of sunlight into sugar. The oxygen absorbed into our lungs is circulated to our cells, allowing us to metabolize sugar into energy, completing the cycle. The energy generated enables us to perform our basic living functions of thinking, moving, digesting, and eliminating. Our minds, fueled by food and oxygen, give rise to the thoughts that contemplate our relationship between local and universal. Breathing intimately connects our cells to the cells of plants, our minds to the mind of God.

The simplest way to access the vitality inherent in the air element is to consciously inhale the fresh breath of plants. Go for a walk in a park or botanical garden. Whenever you are around fragrant or lush vegetation, inhale the life force with your full attention. Imagine the air entering your lungs, being carried to your heart, distributed to your tissues, and fueling your cellular energy centers to support the millions of life processes taking place without your conscious attention. Calculations have shown that with every breath, we take in, on average, one molecule from every breath in our entire atmosphere. Pay attention to the quality of air you breathe and allow your breathing to connect you with all life on this planet.

Fire Energy

The fire element is the expression of light. Einstein elucidated the amazingly spiritual truth that all matter can ultimately be reduced to the interweaving of vibrations. The energy carried by light waves influences everything it touches, catalyzing transformation and metabolism.

We access the fire element through our senses of sight and sensation. The most direct way to consciously connect with the fire in your environment is to put your attention on the sun. Worshiped as divine in Egypt and Babylonia, our local star is ultimately the source of all life on our planet. Allow the light and heat of the sun to infuse you for a few minutes each day. In addition to helping activate vitamin D so we can make stronger bones, focusing on the sun allows us to connect with the incomprehensible power of the universe. Get up early tomorrow and watch the sun rise. Find a beautiful place to watch the sun set. Create rituals to observe the beginning and end of a day on special occasions such as your birthday, your anniversary, or the autumn and spring equinoxes. Honor the quintessential power of the sun.

Water Energy

The water element represents the forces of connectedness and flow. Water cools, nourishes, purifies, and unites. It is the essential element for life that arose in the fluid ocean soup billions of years ago. Our ancestral land hoppers may have taken themselves out of the ocean, but they kept the ocean within them in the form of primitive circulating fluids, which eventually evolved into blood.

We can most directly connect with the water element by spending time in, on, or around natural bodies of water. The healing properties of rivers, springs, and seas have been the stuff of myths since before we invented time. I encourage you to find your nearest pond, lake, stream, river, or ocean and make a regular pilgrimage to it. Allow the cooling, coherent influence of water to calm and soothe your soul. Swim in it, dive into it, sail on it, or simply stand at the shore and observe the flow of the planet's lifeblood as it circulates across time and space, nursing and bathing the earth and all its creatures.

Earth Energy

The earth element represents the densest condensation of space. Atoms held together by invisible cohesive forces give our senses the appearance of stability that we call matter. Expressions such as "solid as the earth" or "the rock of Gibraltar" convey our association of the earth with stability. Mother Earth draws us to her and holds us close, providing us with shelter and sustenance.

How do we access the earth element? Through direct contact. Take off your shoes and socks and wiggle your toes in the grass or sand. Dig your fingers into the ground. Lie down on the ground, close your eyes, and imagine you are hurtling through space on a giant spherical spaceship. Or, as envisioned by the ancients, imagine that the earth is an enormous tortoise on whose back you are riding. Feel the power of the earth as you live and move and acknowledge the abundance she offers. Let's honor her as our mother and she will continue to care for us.

Five Elements, Three Codes of Nature

As discussed in chapter 1, these five Ayurvedic elements represent the primary codes of nature. Although this framework is admittedly simplistic, I have been repeatedly impressed at how useful it remains, despite our sophisticated sciences of chemistry and physics. There is really nothing we can perceive that cannot be considered in terms of these five primary forces. Within an atom we see the space element as the vast emptiness between electrons and protons. The air element manifests itself as the spin of electrons around the atomic nucleus. The fire element is represented by the potential and dynamic energy that exists within every building block of matter. The water element holds matter together through the four forces of gravity, electromagnetism, and the strong and weak nuclear forces. Finally, the earth element is expressed when we see matter as particles rather than as waves of energy. The ancients of both East and West reduced the universe to these five fundamental codes, and although we can look at the world through more complex and sophisticated glasses, there remains an underlying elegance to this timeless model of reality.

In living systems these five primary codes organize themselves into the three mind body elements you now know so intimately as Earth, Fire, and Wind. Each of the three living elements can be transformed by changing the proportion of elements ingested from the world. If you are feeling dull and lethargic (excessive Earth element), seek out more expansion (space) and movement (air), and you will find yourself lightening up. If you are overheating (excessive Fire element), seek out the cooling influence of water or expand your perspective (through space) where there is less oxygen to fuel the flames. If you are experiencing too much turbulence and your mind is racing away from your body (excessive Wind element), seek out the stability of earth and bring in some heat to warm up your body. We are surrounded by nature's medicine in the form of the elements we can access through our senses. Knowing what we are made of and understanding that we are composed of the same stuff that makes the world enables us to imbibe the energy we need to create balance and vitality in our lives.

Enjoy the Planet

Use your senses to ingest vital energy from the environment. Listen to the timeless, primordial sounds of nature. Feel the sensations of the wind, water, and earth on your skin. Open your sense of sight to the vibrations of light. Inhale the aromas of life. Give yourself permission to play outside. Take picnics with your family and friends. Go for bike rides or take a hike. Get into gardening and embrace the rich density of the earth with your fingers. Take a pottery class. Go sailing. Walk barefoot. Play outdoor sports. Use your environment to clear your mind and nourish your spirit.

Making Vital Energy Real

Vital Play

1. Practice connecting with your environment through your senses and the five elements of space, air, fire, water, and earth.
2. Look at the stars, take a walk in the park, feel the sun on your face, play tag with the waves at the shore, wiggle your toes in the grass. Allow the vitality of nature to wash away your cares and infuse your being with life energy.

Delight in What You Have

> I celebrate myself, and sing myself,
> And what I assume you shall assume,
> For every atom belonging to me as good as belongs to you.
> — WALT WHITMAN

Take a piece of paper and write down all the things you are grateful for in your life. Start with superficial things like ATM machines, your dishwasher, and a car that runs. Progress to the more essential components of your life—clean clothes, healthy food, a warm place to sleep. Next, consider the good and fortunate things that have happened to you during your life. Finally, reflect upon the people you have loved in the past or love in the present. Spend a few moments reviewing the gifts you've received throughout your life.

I am grateful for ...

_____

_____

_____

_____

_____

_____

Each day we have the opportunity to celebrate life. Ask someone who is facing a terminal illness, and that person will tell you about the little things that make life worthwhile that they never paid much attention to when they were healthy—the songbirds at dawn, the smell of a baby's hair, the sky at sunset. Experience takes on a quality of enchantment when you do not know how much longer you have to enjoy them.

How do we cultivate this attitude of celebration? There is an Ayurvedic expression that says whatever we put our attention on grows stronger in our life. If we continually focus on what is, or might go, wrong, we'll find ourselves immersed in lamentation. If we focus on what is going well, we'll find ourselves celebrating. Swami Prakashananda tells the classic story of Birbal, the advisor to King Akbar. Birbal was known for interpreting every situation in the best possible light. When envious members of the court told Birbal that the king cut his finger while grooming, Birbal responded in his usual optimistic manner. When the king was informed that his favored counselor was unperturbed by his accident, he became angry and had Birbal thrown into jail.

Later that day while hunting, Akbar lost his way and was kidnapped by a tribe that practiced human sacrifice. Just as Akbar was about to be offered to the gods, his captors noticed his injured finger and decided it was bad luck to sacrifice a wounded offering. Upon his release Akbar thought of his trusted advisor and realized that Birbal had been right again. Arriving back at the palace, the king immediately freed Birbal and begged for his forgiveness. Birbal responded by saying that everything clearly was for the best, for if the king had not thrown him into prison, Birbal would have been on the hunting expedition with the king...and Birbal had no wounds on his finger.

Start paying attention to the little things that go well. The dog did not soil the rug last night. There was less than the usual traffic on the way to work this morning. One of your favorite songs from the sixties was on the radio. You received an unexpected call from a college friend. You got to the store a few minutes before it closed. Your computer did not crash all day. Your spouse was in a good mood when you arrived home from work. Your child got a good grade on her math test today. Your baseball team won the playoff game. Your stock went up. Each time something goes well, celebrate. Each time something goes unexpectedly well, celebrate. Each time something does not go as badly as anticipated, celebrate.

There will always be unanticipated bumps in the road of life. Several years ago a friend of mine required emergency heart surgery while visiting New York City. He was a lifelong vegetarian, never smoked, exercised regularly, and had dedicated his life to spiritual pursuits. When I asked him how he dealt with his sudden life-threatening challenge, he told me he enjoyed his time on the cardiac unit. He enjoyed the opportunity to meditate, read, and dialogue with doctors, nurses, and medical students about the meaning of life. He used a simple metaphor to describe his experience. People enjoy riding roller coasters at an amusement park, confident that although the ride is scary they will return safely to the starting point. In an analogous way, my friend's connection to his inner spirit enabled him to weather and actually enjoy the turbulent ride on which he found himself. Learning to ride out the rough spots and celebrate the smooth patches is key to living a vital life. Use any excuse to transform an experience from ordinary into special. Cultivate an attitude of appreciation and celebration, and your life will feel increasingly magical and vital.

Celebrate Anniversaries of the Heart

Henry Wadsworth Longfellow wrote,

> The holiest of all holidays are those
> Kept by ourselves in silence and apart;
> The secret anniversaries of the heart.

Consider the possible personal events worth celebrating in your life:

- Your birthday
- Your significant other's birthday
- Your mother's birthday
- Your father's birthday
- Your children's birthdays

- Your friends' birthdays
- The day you met your beloved
- The day you moved into your house
- The day you married the love of your life
- The day you left a toxic marriage
- The day you started the job you love
- The day you left the job you didn't love
- The day you started meditating
- And so on …

Make a list of the occasions and milestones that have been significant for you in your life. Include days that brought you joy as well as days that caused you sorrow. Create a personal calendar for yourself that honors the important events of your life and honor the days with rituals of celebration or rituals of release. To commemorate an important event, plant a tree, make a donation, go on a pilgrimage. If you are honoring an occasion of loss, light a candle, write a poem, or release an animal back into its natural habitat. Create ceremonies that capture the essence of the event and celebrate the eternal cycles of nature.

You can celebrate almost anything. The Disney animated version of the Lewis Carroll classic *Alice in Wonderland* showed us how easy it is to find an excuse for a party when Alice, the Mad Hatter, and the White Rabbit held a tea party to celebrate their *un*birthday. Societies create holidays because communities need occasions to break out of their routine, acknowledge their connection to the past, and rejoice in being alive. We can create individual holidays to fulfill a similar personal need.

To recapture that innocent sense of celebration, try playing games with your children. Next time you are driving on a trip, ask your kids to come up with as many new holidays as possible. You will be amazed at their creativity. Children are good at celebrating because they are intimate with their vital energy. They rejoice in the last day of school, the first winter snow, fireflies on a summer night, and fireworks on the Fourth of July because the joy and enthusiasm well up inside and cannot be suppressed. As children we didn't need excuses to play or enjoy ourselves. We considered it our inalienable right to have fun. I know a delightful woman in

San Diego who calls herself a "playologist." Her motto is "Thou shall not commit adulthood." Allow yourself the freedom to be childlike, and vital energy will bubble up in your life. Give yourself permission occasionally to laugh at the world and yourself for how seriously we take things.

Living Fully

We are not going to be here very long. Recognizing this, we have two choices: we can lament the transitory nature of life and become depressed, or we can choose to live the time we have with enthusiasm. I invite you to choose the latter. Celebrate the experience of being human and look for the magical and miraculous in everyday things. Even if there might not be an intended purpose to life according to a cosmic creator, it's still in our best interest to create meaning. Take time to relish the sounds, sensations, sights, tastes, and smells of the world. If you need to be reminded how to be playful look at the young things on the planet—babies, puppies, and kittens. If you genuinely want to experience vitality in your life, reconnect with your passion and enthusiasm by trusting your heart and indulging your deepest desires.

Making Vital Energy Real

Enjoy
1. Make a commitment to find at least one thing to be grateful for each day.
2. Look for excuses to rejoice in your good fortunes, strokes of luck, and blessings in life.
3. Take time on a regular basis to do something just for the sake of enjoyment.
4. Create rituals of celebration that enrich your body, mind, and soul.

Vital Work, Vital Play

One who is serious all day will never have a good time,
while one who is frivolous all day will never establish a household.
—Ptahhotpe, Egypt, 24ᵀᴴ century b.c.

The source of vital energy is not localized in time or space. Rather, it is a state of awareness in which your personalized network of energy and information is plugged into the universal energy generator. In this state of being every action is enriching to your spirit. Most of us glimpse this state when as children we were capable of being completely immersed in the joy of the present moment, unencumbered by thoughts of past or future. Of course, we were also totally reliant on our caregivers, so our happiness was dependent upon the ability of others to fulfill our needs. We moved quickly from glee to gloom if our immediate requirements were not met.

Freedom and responsibility go hand in hand, but as adults we tend to sacrifice freedom at the altar of responsibility. We forget that the reason we chose our positions and possessions in the first place was that we thought they would make us happy. If we are not moving in the direction of increasing lightheartedness, we need to make some different choices. Choose to follow the advice of the twenty-fourth-century b.c. Egyptian philosopher Ptahhotpe, whose quote introduced this section. He said, "Be cheerful while you are alive." Begin today to reestablish joy, enthusiasm, and vitality in your life by creating work and play that are nourishing.

Vital Energy Key #7

Celebrate the Magic of Being

It's good to be just plain happy;
it's a little better to know that you're happy;
but to understand that you're happy
and to know why and how... and still be happy,
be happy in the being and the knowing,
well that is beyond happiness, that is bliss.
—HENRY MILLER, *The Colossus of Maroussi*

People thrive when they are able to create the things they believe
will fulfill their needs and desires. Whether you are cooking a delicious meal, building a new business, or painting a masterpiece,
your fulfillment depends on the creative channeling of your vital
energy. Creativity is the ability to bring into manifestation something that exists only as a result of your attention and intention.
Although needs change at different times of our lives, certain basic desires remain with us for the duration of our time on earth.

We want enough prosperity to have some measure of material freedom. Although we'd probably agree that money alone will not make us happy, having enough affluence to live in a safe house, drive a reliable car, send our kids to college, and go on an occasional holiday is important to most of us living a householder lifestyle. Ayurveda does not make apologies for our need to have a measure of material abundance, recognizing as did the great psychologist Abraham Maslow that we cannot evolve to higher aspirations if we do not have our basic physiological and safety needs met.

We all have a basic need for love. Caring, compassion, trust, acceptance, and a sense of belonging are essential to our experience of happiness and vitality. In the right context, sexual passion as an expression of intimacy can be a gateway to timeless awareness and higher states of consciousness. As we explored in chapter 4, our capacity for intimacy with the faces outside us is proportionate to our capacity to be intimate with the many faces we carry within.

In the last chapter we delved into our need to find meaningful work. Whether this means raising a family, running a business, managing a farm, painting great works of art, helping to heal others, or writing a book, people need to be engaged in meaningful activity that expresses their unique talents. When we are living a life in dharma, we are spontaneously joyful, timeless, and of service.

Material comforts meet the needs of our body. Loving relationships meet the needs of our hearts. Meaningful work meets the needs of our minds. Spirituality fulfills the needs of our souls. In Ayurveda, the word *moksha* describes the state of liberation in which our internal reference point shifts from the individual to the universal. Our connectedness with all beings predominates over our sense of separateness. Our awareness of eternity and infinity transcends our usual limitations of time and space. We live the paradox of being simultaneously cosmic and individual. In this state of awareness, our experience is one of bliss. If ignorance is bliss, then moksha is a state in which we ignore our boundaries in favor of the boundless. Truly, this state of enlightenment is one of wisdom, for the perennial wisdom traditions all point to spiritual freedom as the ultimate goal of humanity. And yet spiritual freedom is not an escape from daily life. Rather, it is the ever-present awareness of the timeless in the midst of time-bound experience. Spirituality is the celebration of the sacred in the thick of daily life. Let's explore how we can be established in unity in the midst of diversity.

Dive within through Meditation

In Psalms we're told, "Be still and know that I am God." In the New Testament, Luke proclaims, "The kingdom of God is within you." From the Upanishads, we learn, "One who meditates and realizes the Self discovers that everything in the cosmos...comes from the Self." In the great Buddhist text, the Dhammapada, we're told, "Like a broken gong, be still and silent. Know the stillness of freedom." Why is meditation so important? It is the only way I know that we can consistently bring our attention to a place that is not trapped by the usual objects of our senses. Most people most of the time are identified with whatever is occupying their mind at the moment. If you are seeing a movie, you become the characters. If you are reading a book, you become the story. If you are watching a television show, you become the program. We lose ourselves in the objects of our perception, sacrificing the experiencer for the experience we are having.

During the practice of meditation, our awareness settles down beyond the usual mental turbulence on the surface of our minds. Rather than flitting from this thought about the past to another about the future, meditation brings us home to the silent expanse of present-moment awareness. The simplicity of the breathing awareness meditation introduced in chapter 5 belies its power. It contains all the basic components of effective meditation processes. Let's review what they are.

The first step of meditation is finding a comfortable spot where you are unlikely to be disturbed. It can be a cozy chair in your den or a supportive pillow on the floor. Although some meditation practices emphasize maintaining an unsupported posture, the purpose of assuming a position in meditation is to allow you to go beyond bodily awareness. If for the entire period of meditation you are thinking about how uncomfortable you are, you are not likely to go beyond a superficial level of physical sensations. On the other hand, I do not recommend you get so comfortable that you fall asleep. For most people, sitting upright in a chair with lower back support is the ideal posture for meditation.

The next step is to find an object of attention that can be used as a vehicle to quiet the mind. This can be in the visual realm, but an inner sound or your breath works best. If you are going to use your breath, simply close your eyes and follow your breathing. Observe the inflow and the outflow of your breath without attempting to alter it in any way. If your breathing speeds up, watch it accelerate. If it slows down, watch it decelerate. However it changes in depth or rhythm, simply allow the changes to occur. With this innocent attitude, you will notice a quieting of your mental activity.

In mantra meditation techniques, including Primordial Sound Meditation as taught at the Chopra Center, a mantra or sound is provided to use as an object of attention. The Sanskrit word *mantra* means "mind instrument," for mantras are tools to hone mental activity. Appropriately used mantras can calm mental turbulence, empower our intentions, and transport us to higher states of consciousness. The classical Vedic mantra "Aum" (often spelled "Om") is held to be the first sound of creation—the cosmic hum. Another commonly used mantra is "So Hum," which is described as the primordial vibration of breath. You can use these mantras effectively, although if you are going to practice mantra meditation, I recommend you receive instruction from a teacher who can choose a sound that is most appropriate for you and guide you in the proper usage of it. Information on locating a qualified meditation teacher is available at the end of the section on sources.

A readily available primordial sound is the sound of your breath. Although it is a subtle distinction from simply observing your breath, another component of breathing meditation is listening to the sound of your respiration. You may hear your breath in your nostrils, your throat, or your chest. Simply follow the sound, making no effort to restrict your breathing. Whenever your mind wanders from the sound of your breath, gently return your awareness to the preverbal flow of wind through your respiratory tree.

Whether you are observing your breath, silently repeating a mantra, or listening to your respiration, you will find that your attention drifts away from the object of attention to another thought in the mind, a sensation in your body, or a sound in your environment. This is a natural part of meditation and cannot and should not be resisted. The most common complaint I hear from newly instructed meditators is that they are having too many thoughts during their practice. The truth is we are always having thoughts, but most of the time we are so engaged in activity that we are not aware of our perpetual internal dialogue. During meditation we begin to notice the subtle but profound separation between our thoughts and the one who is having the thoughts. This early stage of meditation is called "witnessing." Through innocent witnessing of our mental activity, without attempting to manipulate, alter, or resist our thoughts, there is a spontaneous calming of the inner commotion. Any resistance takes us away from the quietness we are seeking, which is the ultimate state of nonresistance.

The next step in the process is the effortless shifting of attention back to the meditation vehicle. Whenever you find that your attention has drifted away from your breath or mantra, gently return it. In this manner, you will find that your thoughts become subtler while you maintain witnessing awareness. At times, you may slip into the "gap" between thoughts and experience awareness without mental activity. This is a "big" experience, for a quiet mind is a rare occurrence for most people, usually associated only with peak experiences. Meditation provides the technology to regularly access this state of "no mind."

If you have ever done scuba diving or snorkeling, meditation will not feel unfamiliar. Unless you are a professional, most people go diving for the sheer joy of being in the present moment. The fish and other sights in the undersea environment are like thoughts during meditation. You notice them and watch them go. Your breathing provides a backdrop for all the experiences you are having. Meditation is diving inside, observing and becoming more intimate with an inner world that is richer and more profound than can be imagined when we are living only on the surface of our minds.

The value of tapping into this expanded domain of awareness is manifold. The experience itself is intensely enjoyable, and just knowing that you can generate this blissful state entirely on your own is empowering. Second, while the mind quiets, there is a corresponding settling of the body, providing a deep rest that is physically rejuvenating. Studies on Transcendental Meditation as well as other practices have suggested that the level of physiologic rest gained during meditation is actually deeper than we usually experience during a night of sleep. The relaxation gained during meditation dissolves fatigue and long-standing stresses. There is an expression in Ayurveda that rest is the nursemaid to humanity; meditation provides a profound experience of rest.

Finally, the regular practice of meditation cultivates awareness of the silence that upholds the vibrations of life, the wholeness supporting the divisions, the eternity underlying the experience of time. Repeatedly diving into the field of conscious energy and then returning to the sensory world leads to an integration of inner silence with the dynamic world of constant transformation. This union of spirit with matter is the essence of spirituality, the essence of bliss, and the essence of vitality. This is sometimes referred to in Eastern traditions as the state of yoga, which means union. It can also be called enlightenment, for when we never lose the undisturbed state of expanded consciousness, even while engaging in our daily thoughts and actions, our identification shifts from individual to universal and we become lighthearted.

Take time to dive within. The usual self-generated obstacles to regular meditation are predictable, depending on the mind body element that is most dominant in your nature. If you are naturally earthy, you may find yourself falling asleep each time you close your eyes to meditate. If you are carrying a lot of fatigue, sleeping during meditation can help to clear away tiredness. However, if you fall asleep every time you sit to meditate, try performing some yoga postures in preparation for meditation to mobilize your vital energy.

If you have a lot of Fire in your nature, your compulsion to finish your work before you are willing to withdraw your senses will be an impediment. It may take a Fire person a while to recognize that meditation is not wasting time; rather, it provides ready access to your deepest source of energy and creativity. You will actually be more productive if you regularly take time to return to your source.

Wind types have the challenge of calming a runaway mind. When Wind people first sit to meditate, they may be overwhelmed by the amount of mental activity they encounter. With practice, meditation brings you beyond the turbulence that keeps you on the surface of your awareness and enables you to dive into the ocean of calm within you. Staying with your practice through the agitation is essential if you are to maintain centered awareness in the midst of incessant change.

If you think you cannot afford the time to meditate, I suggest that you cannot afford *not* to meditate. You'd recognize the fallacy of saying, "I'm too busy driving around all day; I don't have time to go to the gas station to fill my tank with fuel." Similarly, meditation is the time to replenish your physical and emotional reserves so you can have the vitality and dynamism you seek in life. Try meditating twice daily for one month and see for yourself how vitality and bliss permeate your life.

Making Vital Energy Real

Find the Stillness within

1. Take time each and every day to sit and be still. Bring your attention from the infinite world outside to the infinite world inside your own awareness.
2. Become intimate with the silent witnessing presence that transcends the ever-changing objects of your attention. Tap into your inner reservoir of energy and creativity through daily meditation and experience the expansion of bliss and vital energy in all aspects of your life.

Practice Sacred Sex

For many people sex may be their only experience of a blissful state. Deeply wired into our physiology and psychology, sexuality is a primordial force with which nature engages us in her creative process. When sexual energy is flowing through our being, we are vital, open, authentic, and in the moment. If the underlying relationship is loving and respectful, the passion expressed is genuine and nourishing. All of these qualities of sexual intimacy are inherently spiritual.

Throughout the ages, branches of spiritual traditions have recognized the powerful energy of sex that can be channeled for healing and expansion of consciousness as well as for blissful pleasure. Known as Tantra in India and as the Tao of Loving in China, these timeless practices were designed to tap into the connection between lovers to catalyze personal transformation and spiritual evolution. These practices are based on the understanding that raw primordial sexual energy can be channeled upward to fuel personal power, love, and awareness.

Centers of Vital Energy, Centers of Transformation

In its essential form, Tantra identifies seven energy centers in the body, each of which represents a primary layer of life. Known as *chakras* in Sanskrit, the ancient seers envisioned these centers as wheels or vortices of life force. Modern students of Tantra have suggested that these energy zones are metaphors for neural networks or hormonal systems. I have found the consideration of chakras to be most useful as a framework for considering the perennial issues that all of us must address during our lifetimes. Integrating the best aspects of Freud's analytic framework and Abraham Maslow's hierarchy of needs theory, Tantra expounds the understanding that all expressions of life represent the same primal energy. The sex drive, inventiveness, entrepreneurship, artistic creativity, public service, charity, and spirituality are simply the disguises of a universal primordial life force. Learning to tap into the reservoir of this life energy and channeling it to fulfill our aspirations is the goal of Tantra. We can accomplish this through many different approaches, including meditation, chanting, exploration of mythology, yoga, and lovemaking. The network of vital energy pervades our planet, and therefore, we can access the web through any point if we know the right codes. Let's see how we can use the tools of Tantra to develop a conscious connection with our vital energy reservoir.

Our first energy center is at the base of the spine. Known as the root chakra, this center governs our most basic survival needs. When vital energy is moving effortlessly through this center, we have an inherent sense of trust that our basic needs will be met. When this center is congested, we experience core survival anxieties. If we are worried about how we are going to fill our stomachs or have a roof over our head, we are unlikely to think about how we can serve humanity or attain enlightenment.

The second energy center resides in the genital area. When energy is flowing in this chakra, we are in tune with our passion and sensuality. We are comfortable with our sexuality and express our sexual energy in healthy ways. This center is the source of our creative energies that can be used for biological reproduction, the building of enterprises, or the creation of great works of art, depending on how we channel the energy.

The third energy center, localized in the solar plexus, is the seat of our power in the world. When this fiery center is open, our worthy intentions and desires manifest in the world. Congestion in the solar plexus center results in a sense of personal impotence as desires fail to mobilize the energy to orchestrate their fulfillment. Clearing the obstacles from this chakra results in more spontaneous achievement of our goals in life.

The fourth chakra resonates in the heart and embraces the qualities of love and compassion. When vital energy flows effortlessly through this center, we experience nourishing intimacy and loving connectedness to others. The nature of the heart is to overcome separation in time and space. Access to the heart chakra enables us to feel our universality in the midst of diversity. It is the basis of generosity, devotion, and service. Situated at the midpoint between our upper and lower chakras, an open heart center is essential for balance and integration in life.

The fifth chakra resides in the area of the throat, where it governs expression. If this center is blocked, we have trouble expressing ourselves and often feel misunderstood. When the fifth chakra is open and flowing, we spontaneously communicate openly and honestly. People who have issues with this center often complain of the physical sensation of tightness in their throat. Recurrent laryngitis, thyroid problems, and chronic neck pain are often associated with congestion in the throat center. Clearing the obstacles allows us to express our creativity, power, and compassion in the world.

The sixth chakra, located in the forehead, is the center of insight and intuition. Vital energy flowing without restriction through this center nurtures our ability to think synergistically and holistically. We are continuously receiving vast amounts of data about our world that cannot be effectively organized into sequential, linear, causal information. When the sixth energy center is open, we have the ability to synthesize diverse bits of energy and information into a holistic integrated picture. The greatest composers, artists, and scientists across time have intuitively channeled their vital energy into creations and discoveries that express the beauty and wisdom of life.

Finally, the seventh energy center, located at the crown of the head, governs our spiritual journey. When this chakra, known as the "Thousand Petaled Lotus," has fully unfolded, we remember our true nature as divine beings masquerading as human. When all our other layers are clear, open, and resonating harmoniously, we are able to complete our spiritual journey back home to the source of all that was, is, and will be. This is the state of enlightenment and liberation, overflowing with vitality, bliss, and peace.

How do we open the channels of energy so our life force can flow freely? One traditional Tantric approach is to consciously tune the human instrument so it can play a more enlightened song. Each chakra has a primordial sound that can be used to open and clear our vital zones. Using the power of your attention and intention, you can dissolve the impurities that limit the fullest expression of your life force. Sitting comfortably, sequentially bring your attention into each of the major energy centers and sound aloud the mantra for that chakra. Take a deep breath and release the sound as if it was emanating from that place in your body, allowing the sounds to raise your energy level.

Energy Center	Primordial Sound
Base of spine	LAM
Sexual organs	VAM
Solar plexus	RAM
Heart	YAM
Throat	HAM
Forehead	SHAM
Crown	AUM

Making Love Energy

The energy of our sexuality reflects the power inherent in the polarity of life. In traditional Chinese medicine the polar forces are called yin and yang. In Tantra we have Shakti and Shiva. In both these ancient systems, these terms represent the feminine (yin, Shakti) and masculine (yang, Shiva) energies that make the world go 'round. We can enliven these forces to generate greater creativity, vitality, empowerment, and bliss. This requires approaching sex as a sacred exercise rather than merely satisfying a physical appetite. There is a beautiful Tantric vision of the hot, passionate, feminine Shakti energy residing at the base of our spine, and the icy, detached, austere Shiva energy at the top of our head. As the deep, creative, molten earth energy begins to rise, the pure, clear, witnessing, remote ice cap begins to melt. The essence of feminine sensuality and the essence of masculine austerity blend together in the intimate dance of creation, generating wisdom and bliss. Regardless of our sexual or gender identity, each one of us contains both these powerful forces, which are waiting to be awakened.

How can we use these images to spiritualize sexuality? Once again, it is our attention and intention that has transformational power. Approach sex from the perspective of two networks of energy coming together to create a higher, purer vibration. Shift your intention from achieving orgasm to making love, from goal to process. Raise your partner's energies through sounds, sensations, sights, tastes, and aromas. Whisper your appreciation, read inspiring poetry, play beautiful music. Touch, tickle, caress, and tease, using sensitive, creative touch. Create passion-stimulating images. Keep your eyes open while making love, gazing deeply into each other. Watch yourselves in the mirror and enjoy the beauty of your dancing bodies. Indulge in exotic flavors and textures. Use sensuous aromas to engage your memories and emotions. Use all your senses to bring you into the present moment, enlivening vital energy through conscious attention to the sensations in your body.

Your Mind Body Nature and Sex

As is true with every aspect of life, your inherited mind body nature influences your relationship to your sexuality. If you have a preponderance of Earth in your nature, your sexual appetite will generally be steady and consistent. It may take some time to get your desires ignited, but once your energies are flowing, you are a good lover. To connect with your sexual energy it behooves you not to wait until the end of the day to make love, as you may be too drained to mobilize your passions. Look for ways to vary your routine so your lovemaking does not become monotonous—experiment with different places, positions, clothing, aromas, and lighting. Practice mobilizing your sexual energy and using it to vitalize all aspects of your life.

Fire types are naturally passionate, approaching sex with the same voracious appetite with which they pursue other desires. The challenge for Fire lovers is to pace themselves so they can allow the powerful life force to enliven every cell in the body, rather than immediately releasing their heat through orgasm. If you are fiery by nature, practice playing with your sexual energy, allowing it to heat up and then cool down. This sexual fire is the essence of the creative force of the universe. Learning to consciously direct it will invigorate your body, mind, and soul.

Wind types tend to neglect their bodily needs, including their sexual desires. If you have a predominantly windy nature, sex can help to bring you into your body. Sexual energy can be grounding when enlivened consciously. When making love, see how long you can stay with the sensations in your body before expanding to ethereal realms. Keep your eyes open and connect body to body, heart to heart, and soul to soul with your lover. Stay in the present moment and feel the bliss of the vital force pervading your body.

Turn your lovemaking into "for play." The spirit is light-hearted and rejoices in playfulness. Allow yourselves to connect essence to essence at which level you can temporarily transcend your boundaries of individuality. When you physically merge, practice self-referral, staying centered in your own being. Rather than immediately driving toward orgasm, play with the powerful energies you have invoked. Envision vital energy rising from your sexual zone into your heart, flowing into your partner's heart, and circulating between your lower centers and heart centers. When you are about to orgasm, try becoming totally still, seeing if you can retain the energy by bringing it up to your heart. Once you feel some measure of being able to consciously direct the Shakti energy, visualize the energy rising up into the crown of your head. Envision the thousand petal lotus of your crown chakra unfolding as you transform sexual energy into awareness.

This process will dramatically enhance your most intimate relationship as you expand your connectedness with your beloved from physical to emotional to spiritual. Lovemaking at this level becomes mythical as you reenact the primordial exchange of energy that is the basis of creation. For centuries we have tried to separate the material from the spiritual, relegating the body to the profane. As a result, our guilt and ambiguity about sexuality have created a shadowy, disempowering place for sex in modern life, as evidenced by demeaning pornography and the way we use sex to sell everything from cigarettes to automobiles.

I encourage you to view your sexuality as a spiritual gift that can be a blissful tool to integrate body, mind, and soul. Honor your sexuality and use it responsibly. Practice safe sex, recognizing that the powerful energy generated through conscious lovemaking can easily lead to conception. If you are not prepared to invite a new soul into your lives, take the appropriate precautions. With expanded responsibility comes expanded freedom. If you are hoping to create a baby from the interweaving of your love and your genes, there is no better approach than practicing sacred sex. Enjoy the dance of love and watch vitality rise in your life.

Making Vital Energy Real

Vital Sex

1. Make love consciously, using sex to enliven the masculine and feminine forces within your nature.
2. Practice using sacred sex as a technique for exploring deeper emotional and spiritual intimacy.
3. Approach sexuality as an expression of the inherent force of the universe to recreate itself. Channel the energy into higher centers and enjoy the bliss and vitality of being a loving being.

Choose Your Happiness

What is it that brings you joy? What makes you happy? As we have said, there are only two prime motivating forces in life: the pursuit of pleasure and the avoidance of pain. How do we increase the probability that we will drink from the sweet cup of life more often than the bitter? We need to become aware of our choices and how they create the possible event lines that flow from them. Many wise souls have reminded us that if we persist in making the same choices, we are very likely to experience the same outcomes.

What generates the sense of happiness? Although the particular situations and circumstances that create joy are different for each of us, there are basic principles that underlie the experience of delight that we all seek. Let's explore what I call the five "Ls" of happiness—lusciousness, laughter, learning, love, and liberation.

If we look for these sources and invest our time and energy in the pursuit of joy, bliss will blossom in our life.

Offer Luscious Food to All Your Senses

Our senses can be sources of delight. Listening to a Mozart concerto or a Bach suite can elevate the soul, touching the celestial domain. An old Rolling Stones or Beatles album, a great country and western song, or an amazing Miles Davis recording can also bring us into the timeless place where our juices are flowing and we're happy just to be alive. A soothing deep-tissue massage, the fondling by a welcome lover, and the gentle grasp of a baby's hands as she explores your fingers illustrate the potential of our passive tactile sense to evoke tremendous joy. Moving your hands over a piece of bronze sculpture, petting your freshly bathed Irish setter, and molding clay on a potter's wheel reminds us that pleasurable touch can be active as well as receptive.

Watching the sunset over the ocean, viewing a classic movie at home under a warm blanket, taking in the latest Monet art exhibit, walking in a botanical garden, lying on your back gazing at the stars—consider the many ways you can use your visual sense to generate pleasure-inducing chemicals in your nervous system. Beautiful things, both man-made and natural, can bring us gladness as photons of light are transformed in our brains into emotionally pleasing chemicals.

The same holds true for our remaining two senses. The succulent tartness of freshly picked raspberries, the flavorful richness of a home-baked peach pie, the promising sweetness of our first passionate kiss, all have the potential of bringing us to the bliss of the present moment. Finally, the aromas of our world can be uplifting and delighting. For me, the smell of lilacs in the spring transports my soul to some pristine realm of nature where we used to play in the garden of life. The plant kingdom is an abundant source of exhilarating essential oils whose molecules are released into the wind to be dissolved in our nasal passageways. The smells of a puppy's breath, a newborn infant's scalp, and coconut suntan lotion on your child's skin remind us of the richness that pleasurable aromas can bring.

Choose luscious sounds, sensations, sights, tastes, and smells and watch your pleasure meter move toward fullness. It requires a shifting of our attention, which is the smallest quantum of effort. The return on investment is manifold, bringing joy to our body, mind, emotions, and spirit.

Laugh at the World, Laugh at Yourself

As children we laugh for no reason. The bliss of being alive just bubbles up, and we can't control it. If someone asks, "What are you laughing at?" the question itself triggers further rounds of giggling. As we get older, we take ourselves more seriously and need reasons to laugh. A good joke or a comedy movie provides us the opportunity to glimpse the paradox of life, evoking our laughter response. In these days of political correctness, levity has a very restricted place in society, so laughter has been relegated to late-night talk shows, movies, and comedy clubs.

The ego doesn't laugh heartily because it takes itself so seriously. It may chuckle at someone else's tribulations, but it is not comfortable laughing with abandon because the ego needs to stay in control at all times. Our spirit, on the other hand, is the essence of laughter, for seriousness and self-importance are foreign to spirit. Our inner reservoir of energy and creativity masquerades itself in individual expressions but never loses its infinite, timeless essence. As such, the spirit is eternally lighthearted and carefree. This state is the basis of laughter.

Laughter is good for us. Studies from medical centers around the world have suggested that laughter can reduce pain, lower blood pressure, and balance our immune system. A report from Tokyo showed that people suffering with rheumatoid arthritis who listened to traditional Japanese comic stories for one hour had less discomfort, lower stress hormone levels, and improved immune function. A good belly laugh can enhance our immunity for twenty-four hours.

What is funny? With jokes we are led down a path of anticipation until the punch line comes, forcing us to look at the situation in a completely different way. This breaking of the anticipated boundary stops our usual linear thinking, and we experience a burst of joy.

Analyzing or explaining a joke is not funny. The humor is in the unexpected twist that takes us beyond our usual pattern of expectations. The gap that is opened allows for a bubble of bliss to rise to the surface of our awareness, which we experience as laughter. On some level, the whole experience of living life as a human being is hilarious. We take our personal day-to-day trials and tribulations so seriously, knowing all the time that in the overall scheme of the infinite, timeless universe, our frustrations of the day are minuscule. Allow yourself the time and space to laugh. If you have been taking yourself too seriously of late, try spending some time with children or animals. Rent some old Cary Grant comedies, *I Love Lucy* reruns, or *Candid Camera* shows. Seek out the company of people with whom you laugh easily, without meanness, and look for the light side of every life challenge. There are few things that feel as good as a heartfelt laugh. Laughter is a unique expression of the human species. I suspect that it is a gift from the gods.

Keep Learning

Learning something new is joyful. The timeless seers tell us that life is for learning, for when we access new knowledge our minds expand and our souls are nourished. To learn something new we need a willingness to take a risk. If we stay within the boundaries of what is already known to us, we imprison ourselves in the past. The real fun in life happens not when we are reinforcing something that we have known for years but when we are willing to look at things in a new way from a different point of view. When an orthodox medical doctor opens to the possibility of mind body medicine, his worldview shifts and his enthusiasm for healing is rekindled. When a classically trained musician begins exploring jazz, a new harmonic vocabulary becomes available with access to a rich new musical language.

Allow yourself to experience new environments. Look in the newspaper and see what creative performances are available in your town. Go to lectures and seminars that cover topics you are curious about but never found time to delve into before. Try different ethnic restaurants and sample new foods and flavors. Take adult education courses at your local college. Indulge in those piano or painting lessons you have been promising yourself for years. Take a local geology course and learn about the rocks that surround you. Become familiar with the native plants in your region. Learn to identify by sound and sight the birds in your neighborhood. Study the local history of your area. Travel to places slightly off the beaten path and see other ways that people have solved the perennial survival challenges that have faced humanity since the beginning of time.

If you think you already know everything, there is no possibility for learning something new. If you envision yourself as a student of life, you will be in a position to learn something new every day. I encourage you to approach your world with the eyes of a child so you can again enjoy the wonder and magic of the world.

Love with Abandon

The fact we can actually create a word that we use and agree upon to describe the phenomenon of love is a miracle. We use the word in ways that reflect the entire spectrum of human experience. When we tell our children "I love you," we mean we will take care of them until they are ready to take care of themselves. When we tell our lovers in the midst of passion, "I love you," we mean our senses are raging and our partner has what we need to fill our desires. When we say "I love animals," we mean we feel more connected to our environment when other species are in our awareness. When we say, "I love my new car," we mean we like how this object reinforces our self-image. Is there a common thread here?

People, activities, causes, and things we say we love bring us pleasure. They trigger the physiological and chemical cascades that provide the "yum" experience. Things we love physically provide physical pleasure. Those that we love emotionally bring emotional pleasure. Beyond but accessible through both the physical and emotional are those experiences that elicit spiritual pleasure, in which we feel open and connected to the universe. The unifying link between all sources of love is the experience of vital energy flowing. Whether the flow is on a physical, psychic, or transcendent plane, the experience of unrestricted life force feels good. It has been said that the opposite of love is not hate, but rather fear. When we feel apprehensive about opening ourselves, the flow of vital energy is constricted and the pleasure that nourishes us is unavailable. Since we expend a tremendous amount of will keeping ourselves protected from those around us, we spend a lot of life energy keeping our love sequestered.

How do we transform fear into love? The only lasting answer is through the process of self-referral. Maharishi Mahesh Yogi used to say that all love was directed at the Self. "I love you but it's no concern of yours." We love others because they provide us with opportunities to love our Self in other disguises. By Self, of course, I am not referring to our ego-based personality, but rather to our underlying field of awareness—to the realm of spirit. Loving the Self in others is the most selfless act we can perform. In the Upanishads it says:

> It is not for the sake of the husband that the husband is loved, but for the sake of the Self. It is not for the sake of the wife that the wife is loved, but for the sake of the Self.... It is not for the sake of wealth that wealth is loved, but for the sake of the Self.... It is not for the sake of all beings that beings are loved, but for the sake of the Self.

The sensations you feel when you open your heart are yours to keep. It may seem that there is someone or something on the other side upon whom you are dependent for those feelings, but ultimately they're yours. It is the flow that we seek in all our relationships. If you are longing for someone who does not reciprocate your feelings, it is the lack of flow you are grieving in your heart. It is the nature of the heart to want to unify, and obstacles to union are experienced as painful. Knowing what you know about the essential unity of all beings, make the basic assumption that you can love anybody.

Play the game of finding at least one thing to love about every person you encounter. It doesn't have to be major, just something—a gesture, a tone, a smile, a style—something to shift your internal dialogue from judgment and comparison to appreciation and approval.

One of the amazing things about love is that there is no maximum occupancy. Although you may run out of time for all the people you love, you cannot run out of space for more souls to enter your heart. You may have five cats at home, but you can still love another. You may have loved every impressionist painting you have ever seen, but you can still love more. You may already have four grandchildren, but your capacity to love more effortlessly expands if there are more to love. Love, like knowledge, is an amazing commodity; the more you give away, the more you have left. Choose to love generously. Choose to love rather than judge. When you choose love over judgment, you create vital energy that nourishes your heart and soul.

Liberate Your Self

We live on a planet with gravity and, as such, have a tendency to become weighty. And yet bliss results from increasing freedom rather than increasing baggage. We live in a material world and are all subject to the seduction of the sparkly and flashy items that relentlessly cascade across our sensory screen. That new sweater looks so comfortable, that new car so sleek, and that new toy offers so much fun, how could we possibly resist the impulse to call it our own? We all enjoy new things, be they ultrafast 3-D computers, Surround Sound home entertainment systems, or new kitchen appliances. And yet we have all experienced the letdown that occurs when we get what we've been desiring but still feel a little empty.

Not having our desires met is unfulfilling, but having them met rarely provides the lasting happiness we seek. As soon as one need is fulfilled, another rises quickly to take its place. This is the nature of the mind, has always been its nature, and will always be its nature. So what are we to do? We can take a vow to renounce the material world and join a monastery, but most of us will not be happy with this path. The secret again is to be comfortable in the ambivalence. Enjoy your ownership of the material world without letting it own you. Allow things of beauty and utility into your life, enjoy them while they are there, and let them go when it is time to release them.

Before the desire to have something arose in your awareness, you were in a relative state of fulfillment. Once the desire gripped you, you lost your comfort and concluded that the only way for you to feel happy again was to fill the craving. Once the need is satisfied, you return to the initial state of relative fulfillment. The cycle is complete, but you are not really any different from the way you were before the impulse arose in the first place. You go to the shopping mall to buy a birthday present for your friend. While there you see a beautiful cashmere sweater that is perfect for you. You have to have it. A moment ago you were comfortable, but now you are miserable because that sweater holds the key to your happiness. It's outside of your budget, but you decide that you can handle a couple hundred more on your credit card, so you buy it. You get a temporary burst of endorphins as you take possession, returning you to your prior state of contentment. It's not until you are driving home in your car that you begin to have twinges of realization that you didn't really need another sweater and you violated your commitment not to take on more debt. And so you have completed another cycle of desire leading to an action leading to an impression leading to a new desire.

This is the wheel of karma (action) that keeps us tied to the world. How do we escape? We achieve liberation from the cycle of action-impression-desire through awareness. Simply witness the birth and death of desires as they rise and fall in your heart and mind. Bring the process into your conscious awareness and enjoy the perpetual need-creating mechanics of life. Establish the field from which all desires arise as your internal reference point and you will not lose the state of fulfillment while enjoying the

illusion of needing something outside yourself. Focus your attention on your action in the present moment and relinquish your attachment to the fruit of your actions.

In this state you can have anything you want without disturb-
ing your peace. Desires rise and fall like waves on the ocean, but
the ocean is not disturbed by the turbulence. In fact, the movement makes life rich and interesting. While we are alive, we are
not going to lose our desires. The key to vital energy is in enjoying the desires that arise, tapping into the abundant resources of
nature to fulfill our desires, and yet not allowing our essential bliss
to be overshadowed by our desires.

Choose to live a liberating life. Do not allow yourself to get
bogged down with things you don't really need, circumstances
you don't really want to be a part of, or people you don't really
love. When facing a choice or decision, ask if the anticipated outcome will lead to greater freedom and lightness or bondage and
weight. Remember, it is not the job, relationship, person, or situation that gives rise to liberation or confinement; it is your perception and interpretation that creates your reality. Listen to your
mind, feel your heart, and make your choices, realizing that the
inner choice maker who is the source and goal of all choices is already satisfied with the outcome.

Making Vital Energy Real

Cultivate Happiness

1. Make a list of the things that bring you happiness. It may help
   you to think of the five categories, cataloguing those things
   that you find luscious, that make you laugh, that excite you
   about learning, that fill you with love, and that bring you
   freedom.
2. List at least three items in each category so you have a minimum of fifteen things on your list that make you happy. Ask
   yourself when the last time was you allowed yourself to indulge in these joy-producing experiences.

3. Make a commitment to build some time into your schedule to enjoy those things that are enjoyable for you. Decide that you deserve as much happiness as you can create in your life, and begin today to live joyfully.

Strive for Integrity, Embrace Ambiguity

If life were simple, we would each have a clear-cut idea of why we are here with all the instructions on how to fulfill our purpose. If we just followed the plans, we would have the vitality, love, and abundance we seek. Of course life is not simple, and most of us navigate our way through life hoping the choices we make lead to the results we desire. Most of us want to be good people, which means we try to fulfill our needs without hurting others along the way, behaving in ways that are consistent with our words and our beliefs.

To some degree each of us is hypocritical. The only way we can totally avoid being hypocritical is to stop talking, for hypocrisy is the discrepancy between our words and actions. If you acknowledge that you cannot always walk your talk, commit to achieving the highest level of integrity possible. This means establishing the vision of the life you wish to live and aiming to align your words and behaviors with the goals and values you hold important. If you consider yourself to be an environmentalist, recycle your bottles and cans. If you declare that you're a vegetarian, choose not to frequent the local fast-food burger establishment three times a week for lunch. If you believe in animal rights, try to avoid personal care products that are unnecessarily tested on animals.

On the other hand, being in integrity means acknowledging that it is difficult to be a purist, and few causes are well served by a fundamentalist perspective. If you occasionally toss that soda can in the trash because there is not a recycling bin at the airport, it does not mean you have abandoned your values. If despite your best efforts you decide to buy those leather hiking boots to protect your feet, you have not betrayed the cause of animal activism.

Rather, you have accepted the fact that life does not easily arrange itself into neat compartments. The very nature of the life force is its willingness to ooze across rigid boundaries. This is how life moved from the sea to land, across every continent, into every crevice, and to the highest mountaintop. Set the goal and tolerate ambiguity. Do not waste time and energy castigating yourself when you falter. Simply reaffirm your commitment and continue striving for your highest Self.

What is important to you? What are the values you choose to live by? Consider the various realms of life and see if you can define the principles that matter to you.

Vital Environmental Values

What do you hold to be true about your relationship to your environment? What are examples of behaviors that reflect your values?

Example: I believe that it is my responsibility to minimize exploitation of the environment. Behaviors consistent with my beliefs include: (1) riding my bike for short-distance errands; (2) purchasing minimally packaged products whenever possible; (3) bringing fabric carrying bags to the grocery store.

_____

_____

_____

_____

_____

_____

Vital Physical Health Values

What do you hold to be true about your body? What are examples of behaviors that reflect your values?

Example: I believe my body is sacred and that caring for it is a good use of my attention. Behaviors consistent with my beliefs include: (1) ensuring that I eat healthy food prepared with love; (2) taking time to exercise on a regular basis; (3) refraining from intentionally consuming toxic substances.

_____
_____
_____
_____
_____
_____

Vital Emotional Health Values

What do you hold to be true about your relationships? What are examples of behaviors that reflect your values?

Example: I believe that healthy relationships are based on mutual respect and trust. Behaviors consistent with my beliefs include (1) showing up for dates and meetings on time; (2) expressing my feelings openly and honestly; (3) being a good listener when my friends are sharing their vulnerabilities.

_____
_____
_____
_____
_____
_____

Vital Spiritual Values

What do you hold to be true about your spiritual life? What are examples of behaviors that reflect your values?

Example: I believe that a spiritual life reflects an inner dialogue of connectedness to the universe and non-judgment. Behaviors consistent with my beliefs include: 1) meditating every day; 2) spending time appreciating the beauty and wisdom of nature; 3) consciously relinquishing judgment.

_____
_____
_____
_____
_____
_____

A laser beam is more powerful than incandescent light because the wave is coherent. Our intentions are more powerful the more coherent they are with our beliefs and behaviors. Consciously affirm your personal value system; then evaluate your choices in the context of your values. When your actions, words, and beliefs are aligned, your intentions become irresistible. You waste no energy accomplishing your goals, and bliss is your constant companion.

Making Vital Energy Real

Integrate Your Body, Mind, and Soul

1. Bring your values and beliefs into your conscious awareness. Set a vision for your life that is consistent with what you hold to be true and worthwhile.
2. Measure your choices against the vision you have set for yourself. When you find at times that you have drifted away from the values you honor, reset your course, and don't waste valuable vital energy chastising yourself.

Live a Magical Life

For at least four hundred years we have been engaged in a collective argument over which came first, mind or matter. The materialists explain consciousness, thoughts, emotions, inspiration, intuition, love, despair, realization, and ecstasy as the by-products of molecular interactions. From Descartes to Francis Crick, material reductionists hold that the fundamental stuff of the world is matter and all subjective experience is simply a derivative of atoms colliding with each other. Once molecules lose their connectedness to each other in the form of bodies and nervous systems, consciousness evaporates. The materialists argue that our sense of self, memories, ideas, and soul has no existence independent of matter.

On the other side of the argument are the vitalists who argue that spirit is the essential stuff of creation, with matter a by-product of consciousness. Mind is primary, matter is secondary. Consciousness conceives, governs, and becomes the material world. The same place nature goes to create a molecule, our minds go to create a thought. The physical world is just an illusion of condensed consciousness perceived by consciousness through the self-generated apparatus of a nervous system.

At first consideration, these viewpoints seem irreconcilable. We have experienced the division of consciousness and matter taken to the extreme in medicine, where materialists attempt to explain all behavioral phenomena including disease in terms of genetics and biochemistry, while mind body proponents advocate that our attention and intentions can directly alter the molecules of our body.

I suggest that these perspectives are really not so opposed. It is the nature of the universe to evolve through contrast, and the mind/matter argument is simply another construct of the mind doing what it does best—creating divisions of the indivisible. Can anyone really argue that without a physical nervous system I would have difficulty communicating these thoughts? And without these thoughts, where would the concept of matter or molecules arise? If the capacity for molecules to organize into life forms is inherent in the substance of matter, what an amazing demonstration of intelligence in the universe! And if the entire physical creation is ultimately a dream of Lord Vishnu floating on the cosmic ocean of eternity, what an amazing illusion we collectively hallucinate. The ultimate expression of reverence for an invisible intelligent creator may be the scientific belief that God did such a good job of establishing the laws of nature that His or Her presence is no longer necessary. Whether we believe that our minds emerge from molecules or that our molecules emerge from the mind, the world is a truly miraculous creation.

Reality is an act of selective perception and interpretation. We are living in a scientific age and are conditioned to see the world through the window of a scientific perspective. Personally, I find the scientific paradigm fascinating and nourishing, but like all points of view, science is limited by what it conceives of as possible. When the prevailing model of reality cannot adequately explain our experiences, a new, more expanded one will replace it. What might this new vision offer? I see it encompassing both the facts and the magic of life. It will embrace both the linear, rational pathways of thought and the synergistic, intuitive, mythical realms of experience. We cannot live a vital life without the sparkle of mystery.

How do we awaken the magic within us in order to engage with the magic that surrounds us? We live our lives as mythical adventures. Each of us is on a personal quest, recapitulating the perennial human drama. We can raise our personal journey to a universal level by identifying with the eternal stories of life. Throughout humanity individuals have connected with their ancestors and their world through mythological legends, the essential threads that weave us into the eternal fabric of life. The symbols we invest with power and the stories we tell generation after generation nourish our souls in unparalleled ways. Disconnected from our collective magic, life is bland and uninspiring. Plugged in to our mythical world, we rise to heroic status and at times we can ascend to divinity. Our inner symbols are powerful sources of vital energy.

"Once upon a time..." "Long, long ago in an ancient place..." Just these few words of introduction transport us to realms beyond time and space. They allow us to access the collective domain of our souls where all love is romantic, all quests heroic, and all failures tragic. In every culture around the globe since the beginning of tribal time, people have wrapped themselves in the stories of their land and ancestors, protecting themselves from isolation and mortality. A connection to mythology empowers and revitalizes both the individual and the community.

Although myths are interwoven into the very substance of the human psyche, our modern cultural myths have not served us well. Humankind has traditionally used symbols and stories to connect us with our land and our progenitors, but modern people are generally alienated from both. Urban gangs and religious cults are unhealthy efforts to create mythical connections. We attempt to tap into a collective adventure through our media in mythical projections such as *E.T.* or *Star Trek*, but in general, we've become detached from our archetypal vitality.

What can we do to reconnect? We need to recapture our connection with an enchanting world. Get to know the land you are living on. What nature spirit did the native people recognize in a nearby mountain or stream? Where are the local power spots? What feelings are invoked in you as you explore the land on which you live? Become acquainted with the trees, birds, and animals in your community. Introduce yourself to the dogs and cats in your neighborhood. Become familiar with the constellations in the night sky and learn the stories that have been told about them for ages.

The great explorer of our mythical realms, Joseph Campbell, told Bill Moyers in *The Power of Myth*, "People say that what we're all seeking is a meaning for life. I don't think that's what we're really seeking. I think that what we're seeking is an experience of being alive, so our life experiences on the purely physical plane will have resonances within our own innermost being and reality, so that we actually feel the rapture of being alive. That's what it's all finally about, and that's what the clues help us to find within ourselves."

These clues that we're part of something much bigger than our ordinary reality provide us with the power to live a vital life. The mythical warrior Don Juan Matus told Carlos Castaneda, "Human beings have a very deep sense of magic. We are part of the mysterious. Rationality is only a veneer with us. If we scratch that surface, we find a sorcerer underneath."

Those moments when we experience the parting of the veil provide us glimpses into the unfathomable organizational power of the universe. At the very moment you gain insight into an agonizing dilemma, the sun bursts from behind a cloud, bathing you in warmth and light. Struggling with a vocational decision, you are about to surrender to despair when an old friend calls you with the opportunity of a lifetime. You wonder if you will ever again find love when you chance upon a beautiful being under the most improbable circumstances. You feel depressed and alienated from life until, while hiking, you unexpectedly cross paths with a family of deer, rekindling your sense of wonder and appreciation for nature's gifts. These moments fill us with enthusiasm and vital energy as they remind us of the magic and mystery behind the scenes.

Be alert to the omens that make life mystical. You cannot see the magic if you do not allow for its possibility. When you encounter something outside of your usual routine, pay attention and allow the wonder of the improbable to awaken you. Do not be afraid to endow the ordinary with delight. Be open to dreaming the collective dream that has the power to awaken humanity. Notice the rainbows, the phases of the moon, and shooting stars. Be awake to the symbols that serve as vehicles to the mythological domain. See the deeper meaning in the icons of Western spirituality—the crucifix, Star of David, angelic beings—and do not allow yourself to be limited by the narrow interpretations suggested by divisionist theology. Read the stories of heroes and heroines, allowing your imagination to resonate with archetypal forces. Align yourself with others who see themselves on a mystical journey and overcome your resistance to being extraordinary. A mystical life is rich in vital energy.

The greatest gift of being human is the freedom to make choices. I encourage you to choose a magical life, filled with mythology, mysticism, and mystery. This is the path to vital energy, inspiration, creativity, and bliss. This is the path to a life worth living.

Postscript

Embracing Vital Energy

Ever since Happiness heard your name,
It has been running through the streets
trying to find you.
—Hafiz

The word *vital* is derived from the Latin root "vita," which means life. Vital energy is the energy of life, that miraculous organizing principle of molecules and forces that orchestrates its own evolution through learning and creativity. Vital energy is the most primordial force of nature, driving the universe toward conscious awareness of its own existence. Over billions of years of evolutionary time, atoms have organized into molecules, molecules into complex chemicals, and chemicals into self-reproducing entities. Since the genesis of life more than four billion years ago, single cells have evolved into increasingly complex life forms. With the dawning of humanity sometime within the last one hundred thousand years, nature has created a remarkable instrument—the human nervous system capable of being in awe of itself.

To be overflowing in vital energy is to be aligned with the infinite, eternal creative force of the universe. It is a state of being in which we have unlimited access to the field of unbounded energy deep within our nature. The paradox of vital living is that we need to go beyond the boundaries of our personal individuality in order to generate personal power. Immersing ourselves in the mythical domain brings enchantment to our worldly endeavors. Immersing ourselves in the universal domain brings the energy of the boundless into each of our acts performed within the boundaries of time and space.

Each day in my practice I see people struggling and suffering because their access to their own vital energy is blocked. This book arose from my need to understand why some people are inexhaustibly energized while others are chronically fatigued. I learned that energy depletion could be due to problems at many different levels. For some people, their lack of energy is primarily a physical problem. For them, a better diet, nutritional supplements, or a physical exercise program may provide the invigorating boost they require.

For others, the obstacles to vitality exist on a subtler level. Emotional clarity, nourishing relationships, and meaningful work are needed to get their juices flowing. They must reduce their tolerance for toxicity, be it toxic substances, emotions, or relationships, in order for vital energy to flow.

For all of us, the most important journey is the one that carries us back home, restoring our connection with our source of vital energy. From the moment that the first atoms joined together, life has been on a sacred quest to achieve unity above separation. The closer we approach the source, the greater access we have to the vital treasure house that resides there. Each key described in *Vital Energy* brings us closer to the inner sanctum of energy, creativity, and joy.

In the beginning light emerged out of the void. In essence we are stardust, born at the time of the primordial nova. We are beings of light in a vast universe of light. In essence, we are vital energy.

Sources

Introduction

Spierings, E., M.J. van Hoof. Fatigue and sleep in chronic headache sufferers: an age- and sex-controlled questionnaire study. *Headache* 37 (1997):549–552.

    In this study from the Brigham & Women's Hospital in Boston, 60% of controls and 70% of headache sufferers reported fatigue.

Cox, B., M. Blaxter, et al. The health and lifestyle survey. London: *Health Promotion Research Trust* 1987:61–62.

    In this 1987 report from England, 20% of British adults reported they "always felt tired" during the preceding month.

Key 1: Seek Your Self

Recommended General Reading

Chopra, D. *Perfect Health*. New York: Harmony Books, 1991.

Frawley, D. *Ayurvedic Healing*. Salt Lake City: Passage Press, 1989.

Simon, D. *The Wisdom of Healing*. New York: Harmony Books, 1997.

Key 2: Clear Your Toxins, Digest Your Past

Murchie, G. *The Seven Mysteries of Life*. Boston: Houghton Mifflin Company, 1978.

    This book is filled with fascinating information on the dynamic nature of life.

Brooks, S.M., L. Benson, and M. Gochfeld. Types and sources of environmental hazards. In *Environmental Medicine*, S.M. Brooks, et al., eds. St. Louis: Mosby, 1995, p. 12.

    The quantity of chemicals released into our environment as described in this scholarly work is startling, distressing, and motivating.

Environmental Protection Agency Web site. 1998. Twenty-five years of environmental progress at a glance. www.epa.gov

    For the latest EPA challenges and information, check out this user-friendly Web site.

Key 3: Feed Your Body, Nourish Your Soul

Le Pars, P.L., M.M. Katz, et al. A placebo-controlled, double-blind, randomized trial of an extract of *Ginkgo biloba* for dementia. North American EGb Study Group. *JAMA* 278 (1997):1327–1332.

This study on patients with dementia demonstrated that Ginkgo biloba in doses of 120 milligrams per day helped to stabilize or improve their cognitive function.

Chen, X. Cardiovascular protection by ginsenosides and their nitric oxide releasing action. *Clinical and Experimental Pharmacology and Physiology* 23 (1996):728–732.

This laboratory study from China is the first to suggest a mechanism to explain ginseng's reputation as a natural sexual performance enhancer.

Siegel, R.K. Ginseng abuse syndrome. *JAMA* 241 (1979):1614–1615.

Fourteen out of 133 people taking an average of 3 grams of ginseng root experienced elevated blood pressure, nervousness, sleeplessness, skin rashes, and morning diarrhea.

Linde, K., G. Ramirez, et al. St. John's wort for depression—an overview and meta-analysis of randomized clinical trials. *BMJ* 313 (1996):253–258.

This analysis of twenty-three clinical trials found that hypericum was more effective than placebo, as effective as standard antidepressant drugs, and had a low incidence of side effects.

Meydani, S.N., M. Meydani, et al. Vitamin E supplementation and in vivo immune response in healthy elderly subjects. *JAMA* 277 (1997):1380–1386.

A study of 88 adults over the age of 65 who took 200 milligrams per day of Vitamin E had significant improvements in indexes of immune function.

Key 4: Release Depleting Emotions, Cultivate Love

Gibran, K. *The Prophet.* 1923. New York: Alfred A. Knopf, 1923, p. 32.

Recommended General Reading

Ford, D. *The Dark Side of the Light Chasers.* New York: Riverhead Books, 1998.

Goleman, D. *Emotional Intelligence.* New York: Bantam Books, 1995.

Smith, T.J. *Full Share.* Tucson, Ariz.: Whitewing Press, 1995.

Key 5: Move to Nature's Beat

Recommended General Reading

Douillard, J. *Body, Mind, and Sport.* New York: Crown Trade Paperbacks, 1994.

Key 6: Work with Meaning, Play with Passion

Prakashananda, S. *Don't Think of a Monkey.* Fremont, Calif.: Sarasvati Productions, 1994.

This delightful book contains many rich teaching stories.

For information on programs to keep you from taking life too seriously contact: Kyle Katz at Playology, Inc., 2707 Oceanfront Walk, San Diego, CA 92109. Phone (619) 488-7400.

Recommended General Reading

Blank, W. *9 Natural Laws of Leadership.* New York: Amikon Books, 1995.

Klein, E. and J.B. Izzo. *Awakening Corporate Soul.* Lions Bay, British Columbia: Fair Winds Press, 1998.

Secretan, L.H.K. *Reclaiming Higher Ground.* Toronto: Macmillan Canada, 1997.

Key 7: Celebrate the Magic of Being

Wallace, R.K., H. Benson, A.F. Wilson. A wakeful hypometabolic state. *American Journal of Physiology* 221 (1971):795–799.

>In this groundbreaking paper, practitioners of meditation are shown to elicit unique physiological changes.

Campbell, J. *The Power of Myth.* New York: Doubleday, 1988, p. 5.

>This beautiful book from which the quote on page 239 is taken is a must-read for any mythical explorer.

Castaneda, C. *The Power of Silence.* New York: Washington Square Press, 1987, p. 167.

>Castaneda's exploration of a magical world with the Mexican Indian sorcerer Don Juan Matus opened our minds and souls to the possibility of alternative realities.

Recommended General Reading

Anand, M. *The Art of Sexual Magic.* New York: Jeremy Tarcher/Putnam, 1995.

Bulfinch, T. *Bulfinch's Mythology.* New York: Modern Library, 1993.

Dunas, F. *Passion Play.* New York: Riverhead Books, 1997.

Easwaran, E. *The Upanishads.* Tomales, Calif.: Nilgiri Press, 1987.

Hamilton, E. *Mythology.* New York: Meridian, 1989.

Johari, H. *Tools for Tantra.* Vermont: Destiny Books, 1986.

Kinsley, D. *Hindu Goddesses.* Berkeley: University of California Press, 1986.

Woolger, J.B. and R.J. Woolger. *The Goddess Within.* New York: Fawcett Columbine, 1987.

Vital Energy Enhancing Suggestions

These are a few books that have enhanced my vital energy. They are offered in love and friendship.

Castaneda, Carlos. *The Power of Silence*, Pocket Books, 1991.

Chopra, Deepak. *How to Know God*. Random House, NY, 2000.

Dass, Ram. *How Can I Help?* Knopf, 1985.

Easwaren, Eknath. *The Upanishads*. Nilgiri Press, Tomales, CA, 1987.

Ford, Debbie. *The Dark Side of the Light Chasers*. Riverhead Books, NY, 1998.

Fox, John. *Poetic Medicine*. Jeremy P. Tarcher/Putnam, NY, 1997.

Hagen, Steven. *Buddhism Plain and Simple*. Broadway Books, 1998.

Ladinsky, Daniel. *I Heard God Laughing—Renderings of Hafiz*. Sufism Reoriented, Walnut Creek, CA, 1996.

Osho. *Meditation: The First and Last Freedom*. St. Martins Press, 1997.

Robbins, Tom. *Jitterbug Perfume*. Bantam Books, 1990.

Venkatesananda, Swami. *The Concise Yoga Vasistha*. State University of New York Press, Albany, NY, 1984.

Recommended Audiotapes

Borysenko, Joan. *The Ways of the Mystic*. Hay House, 1999.

Chopra, Deepak. *Ageless Body, Timeless Mind*. Nightingale-Conant, 1993.

Chopra, Deepak and David Simon. *Training the Mind, Healing the Body*. Nightingale-Conant, 1998.

Gawain, Shakti. *Living in the Light*. Nataraj, 1993.

Myss, Caroline. *Anatomy of the Spirit*. Sounds True, 1996.

Thurman, Robert. *Making the World We Want*. Audio Wisdom, 1998.

Index

abundance, 13–14
abundance consciousness, 193
acceptance, 195–196
acetic acid, 85
addictive behavior, 67
ADORE (Accept, Demonstrate, Open, Receive, and Express), 195–199
adrenaline, 65
agni, 76, 77, 78
Ahhhh breath, 163–164
air energy, 201, 203
Al-Bistami, Abu Yazid, 13
alcohol, 66, 67
Alexander the Great, 7, 8
allyl cysteine, 89, 90
aloe vera, 86
Alzheimer's disease, 102
ama, 9–10, 103
American vegetarian meal, 86–87
antioxidants, 65, 89, 90, 108
appetite
    and mind body type, 81–83
    importance of, 76–78
    listening to, 78–79
    rekindling, 80
appetite gauge, 79
Aristotle, 113
aromas, as therapy, 62
ascorbic acid, 85
ashwagandha, 100–101, 106
asparagus, 86
astringent, 86, 93

atherosclerosis, 110
awareness. *See* meditation
Ayurveda, 9, 18

Bacopa monniera. See Brahmi
balance
    achieving, 39–40, 42, 43, 44
    emotional, 124–130
bananas, 86
basic needs, 13–14
bathing, 155
beans, 86, 92
beliefs, 50–51, 52–53
Bellows breath, 162–163, 164
Benson, Lynette, 55
berries, 89
beta-carotene, 65, 108–109
Bhagavad Gita, 168
Bible, 14
bioflavonoids, 89, 90
biological rhythms, 151–160
Birbal, 206
bitter taste, 80, 86, 92, 93
bliss sheath, 49–50, 52
Brahmi, 101–102, 106
breakfast, 156
breathing, 160–164, 201
    abdominal, 161–162
    empowering, 163–164
    energizing, 162–163
    in meditation, 214–215
breathing awareness meditation, 155–156
broccoli, 86, 89, 96

Web site Announcement

If you have enjoyed this book and wish to learn more about ways to enhance your health, vitality, and personal development, please visit our new Web site: www.MyPotential.com.

For Further Information

To locate a Chopra Center for Well Being-certified Primordial Sound Meditation Instructor (to learn meditation) or a certified Creating Health Educator (for courses applying the principles of Ayurveda to enhance well being), please call toll-free (888) 424-6772 or visit our Web site at www.chopra.com and open our Directory of Instructors page.